Honey, WHAT DO WE GOT?

Honey, WHAT DO WE GOT?

A Week-By-Week Pregnancy Cookbook

Rachael & Tom Sullivan

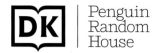

Publisher Mike Sanders
Art & Design Director William Thomas
Editorial Director Ann Barton
Editor Brandon Buechley
Designer Becky Batchelor
Creative Team Chanelle Smith-Walker, Hristina & Bryant Polk, Jessi Lancaster and Ally Rabon
Recipe Tester Ashley Brooks
Proofreaders Christina Guthrie, Lisa Himes
Indexer Celia McCoy

First American Edition, 2025
Published in the United States by DK Publishing
1745 Broadway, 20th Floor, New York, NY 10019

The authorized representative in the EEA is Dorling Kindersley
Verlag GmbH. Arnulfstr. 124, 80636 Munich, Germany

Copyright © 2025 Meals She Eats
DK, a Division of Penguin Random House LLC
24 25 26 27 28 10 9 8 7 6 5 4 3 2 1
001–342696–FEB2025

A catalog record for this book
is available from the Library of Congress.
ISBN 978-0-5938-4635-3

DK books are available at special discounts when purchased in bulk for sales promotions, premiums, fund-raising, or educational use. For details, contact SpecialSales@dk.com

Printed and bound in Italy

www.dk.com

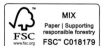

MIX
Paper | Supporting responsible forestry
FSC™ C018179

This book was made with Forest Stewardship Council™ certified paper – one small step in DK's commitment to a sustainable future.
Learn more at
www.dk.com/uk/information/sustainability

DEDICATION

To our sweet Rosie—

You are a bright light in our lives. Always know how deeply you are loved, how special you are, and how much joy you bring to everyone who meets you. We can't wait to see the beautiful story you'll write in this world.

To Lenore—

Mom, you helped grow our family closer than we were ever able to explain to you. We miss you dearly but think about you daily.

For all the moms who have loved and lost—

The brave, the strong, and the endlessly loving. To those who have carried a child in their hearts instead of their arms, your love is real, your grief is valid, and your strength is immeasurable. May you find comfort in knowing that you are never alone, and that the love you hold for your little one is a light that will never dull.

CONTENTS

There's Always a Reason to Celebrate......................................10
Our Fertility Journey...14
How This Book Came to Fruition 20
Week-By-Week Size Chart..22

FIRST TRIMESTER

week 8

Blueberry Skillet Pancake...30
Lemon, Blueberry & Lavender Overnight Oats...........................33
Blueberry & Chipotle Chicken 34

week 9

Raspberry Ginger Tea...37
Raspberry Dijon Chicken...38
Raspberry Marmalade Breakfast Sliders................................... 41

week 10

Cherry Vinaigrette Wedge Salad...42
Cherry-Balsamic Brussels Sprouts..45
Cherry & Rosemary Chicken 46

week 11

Arugula & Fig Pizza...49
Fig & Walnut Cornbread..50
Fig & Banana Smoothie...53

week 12

Key Lime Pie Overnight Oats...54
Spicy Margarita Mocktail.. 57
Cilantro-Lime Coconut Chicken...58

SECOND TRIMESTER

week 13

Grilled Peach-Basil Goat Cheese Sandwiches............................66
Lamb with Peach & Mint Pesto..69
Peach-Cobbler Cookies..70

week 14

Pear-Mostarda Pork Chops 73
Pear & Prosciutto Poppers 74
Fall-Winter Pear Salad 77

week 15

Apple Nachos 78
Apple, Sweet Potato & Sausage Breakfast Skillet 81
Green Apple BLT 82

week 16

Avocado Huevos Rancheros Toast 85
Mint Chocolate Chip Avocado Ice Cream 86
Mediterranean Chickpea Avocado Boats, Three Ways 89

week 17

Endive Cups, Three Ways 90
Endive Stir-Fry with Vegetables & Ground Turkey 93
Grilled Endive with Fig, Apple & Walnut Salad 94

week 18

Pomegranate Quinoa Salad 97
Lemonade with Pomegranate & Rosemary Ice Cubes 98
Pomegranate & Dark Chocolate Bites 101
Pomegranate-Stuffed Sweet Potatoes 102

week 19

Mango & Beef Skewers 105
Mango Smoothie Bowl 106
Chocolate-Covered Dried Mangos 109

week 20

Dragon Fruit & Shrimp Poke Bowl 110
Pink Drink 113
Dragon Fruit Kabobs 114

week 21

Sweet Potato Shepherd's Pie 117
Sweet Potato Gnocchi 118
Sweet Potato Toast, Three Ways 121

week 22

Candied Grapefruit Parfait 122
Fish Tacos with Grapefruit Avocado Salsa 125
Rosemary Grapefruit Granita 126

week 23

Banana Sushi, Three Ways 129
Banana French Toast 130
Banana Recovery Smoothie 133

week 24

Carrot Ribbon Salad 134
Ginger Carrot Soup 137
Carrot Fries with Dipping Sauce 138

week 25

Charred-Corn Maque Choux 141
Charred Corn & Onion Chowder 142
Thai Street-Corn Salad 145

week 26

Jicama Ceviche with Jicama Chips 146
Sautéed Shrimp with Jicama & Cilantro Slaw 149
Jicama Fries with Creamy Avocado Dipping Sauce ...150

THIRD TRIMESTER

week 27

Roasted Grape & Red Onion Pork 158
Sonoma Chicken Salad 161
Grape Harvest Crisp 162

week 28

Cucumber Tahini Salad 165
Cucumber Salsa Verde with Shrimp 166
Mediterranean Cucumber Wrap 169
Cucumber Margarita Mocktail 170

week 29

Crispy Eggplant Tacos 173
Eggplant Dip 174
Eggplant Lasagna Stack 177

week 30

Coconut Curry Chicken & Vegetables 178
Coconut-Crusted Seafood 181
Piña Colada 182

week 31

Jibarito Chicken Sandwich 185
Broiled Plantain Ice Cream Split 186
Tostones with Herb Dipping Sauce 189

week 32

Cuban Slaw 190
Cabbage Stir-Fry 193
Stuffed Cabbage Rolls with Tomato Sauce 194

week 33

Cauliflower Steak with Chimichurri..............................197
Cauliflower Curry...198
Blackened Cauliflower...201

week 34

Pineapple Whip 202
Shrimp Fried Rice in a Pineapple Boat.........................205
Slow-Cooker Pineapple Pulled Pork, Three Ways.................206

week 35

Roasted Butternut Squash Soup 209
Chipotle Butternut Squash & Plantain Bowl.....................210
Sheet Pan Butternut Squash & Lemon Cashew Yogurt........213
Butternut Squash Risotto......................................214

week 36

Grilled Prosciutto-Wrapped Cantaloupe.........................217
Yogurt Toast with Cantaloupe Ribbons 218
Cantaloupe & Herb Salad.......................................221

week 37

Rhubarb-Glazed Chicken Wings..................................222
Crispy Duck Breast with Rhubarb Chutney 225
Rhubarb, Apple & Almond Cobbler...............................226

week 38

Kale Caesar Salad...229
Baked Kale Frittata...230
Kale Chips, Four Ways...233

week 39

Savory Pumpkin Pasta Sauce....................................234
Pumpkin French Toast Casserole 237
Pumpkin Oatmeal 238
Pumpkin Hummus 241

week 40

Watermelon Poutine 242
Watermelon Salad 245
Watermelon "Cake" 246

The Fourth Trimester 248
Index...250
Acknowledgments...255
About the Authors...256

THERE'S ALWAYS A REASON TO CELEBRATE

Honey... congratulations on your pregnancy! And welcome to the next chapter of your life. We have a lot to celebrate!

Whether you conceived on the first try or faced the challenges many experience on their journey to pregnancy, it's undeniable that the process is complex and at times overwhelming. The extensive list of factors involved in actually getting pregnant highlights just how much must align perfectly for conception to occur. Even under ideal conditions, getting pregnant can take time, sometimes even years. Given all this, we believe that successfully becoming pregnant is a significant achievement, one that deserves to be celebrated often!

For us, becoming pregnant and growing our family was a monumental milestone—something we did not take for granted. We wanted to be intentional about pausing and appreciating this season in our lives. As life sped up around us, we made a conscious choice to slow down and celebrate every step of this journey. In our family, celebrating often means cooking up delicious food and enjoying it together or with loved ones.

These milestone celebrations not only sparked meaningful conversations, but also anchored us in the moment. Yes, life was changing—a new chapter is beginning—and not every moment would be filled with sunshine and rainbows . . . but we chose to *celebrate anyway.*

There will be a lot of traditional milestones you will celebrate. The day you walk into your first prenatal appointment, hear your baby's heartbeat, and see the baby growing inside of you. You'll celebrate by telling your friends and family you're expecting and watching their reactions, which will become core memories for the rest of your life. You'll find out the baby's sex or decide to keep it a surprise! You'll purchase a maternity pillow, feel your baby move, and others will be able to feel your baby move . . . the most surreal feeling in the world (that is until they start kicking you in the ribs come the third trimester). You may celebrate with family and friends in the form of a baby shower. You'll purchase your first baby item, assemble a nursery, and nest. Feeling labor pains is something to celebrate as well, because it means that soon enough you get to meet your baby and see who they are.

Aside from the joyous milestones, there will be a lot of tough milestones for you as well, ones that don't feel as celebratory in a traditional fashion. You may be a part of the morning sickness crowd, which—let's be honest—isn't reserved for just the mornings. You may experience food aversions, causing your stomach to turn in an instant. You'll inevitably outgrow your clothes and fight the battle between buying maternity clothes, sizing up, or trying to survive with a rubber band to expand a few inches in your waistline to make it more comfortable. You will cry. Whether it's because you watched an emotional video about a lost dog finding his way home, you were placed on another daycare waitlist, or your body is swelling in places you didn't think possible. Your hormones will be a fun adventure, and one you will have to navigate every day. Strangers will inevitably comment on your weight, "you look so small" or "you look like you're about to pop," and I know these comments may make you want to pop them in the face from time to time. There may also come a time when you can't pick something up off the floor or see your feet anymore.

All of this is to say that pregnancy has its beautiful and not-so-beautiful moments . . . but celebrate *anyway*. As a parent, you will learn that it can be difficult to capture the beauty in everyday moments. By definition, there is no "perfect pregnancy" because that implies that it has no flaws or limitations. Every aspect of your pregnancy will have its own unique beauty and significance. Be it the good days or the bad ones, these moments will shape you, teach you, and ultimately, bring you closer to the parent you are going to be.

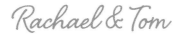

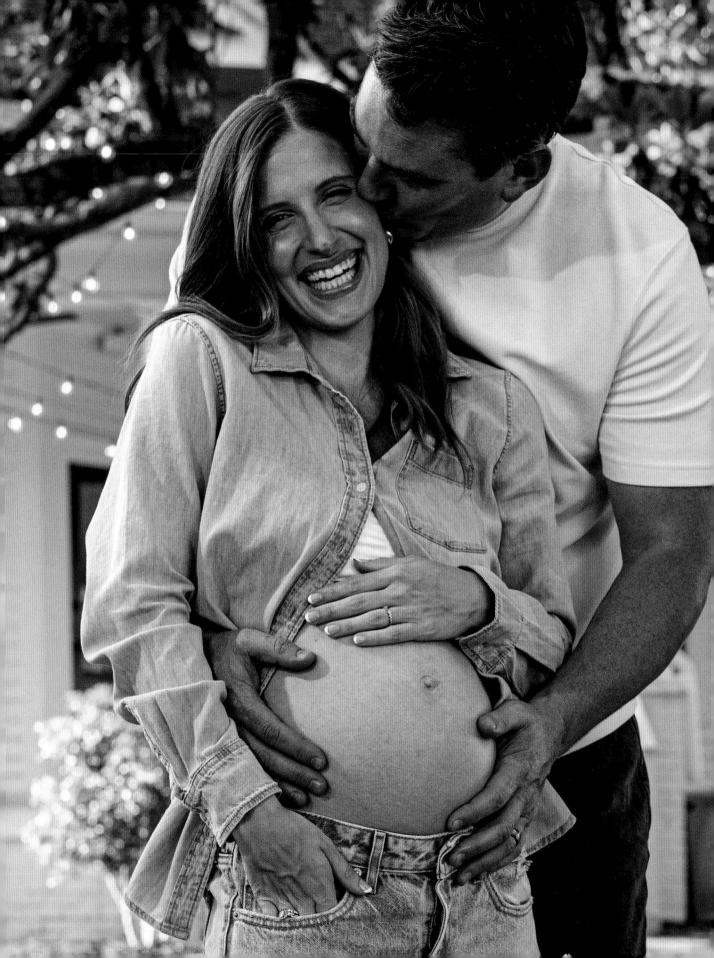

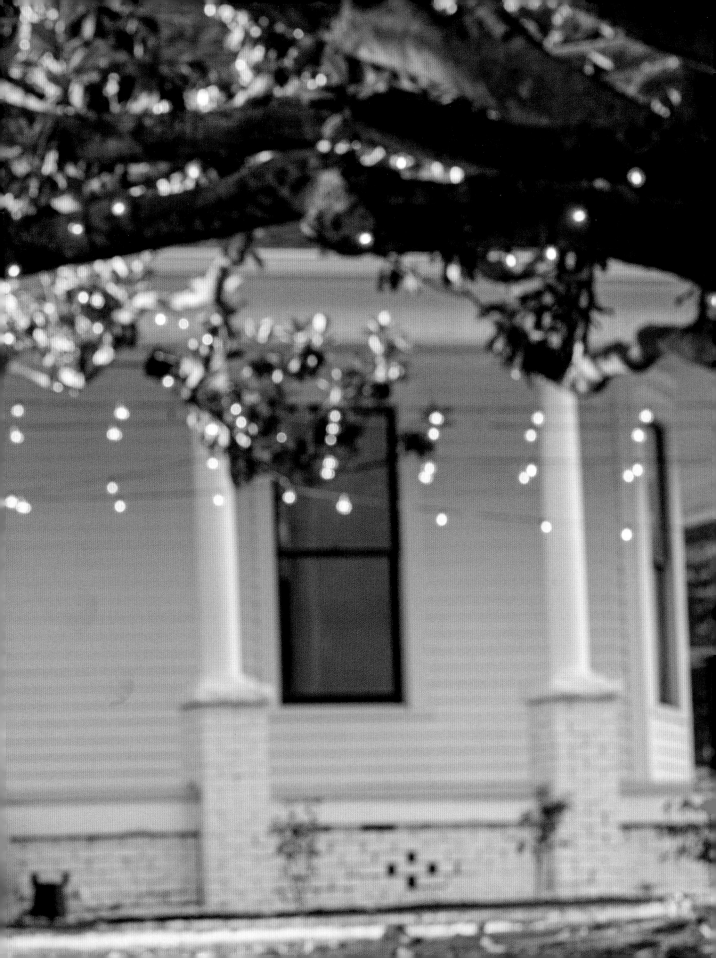

OUR FERTILITY JOURNEY

Life is a never-ending roller coaster of ups and downs, ebbs and flows, and highs and lows. This translates to every aspect of your life. Whether it's your relationships, your work, your mental, physical, and emotional health, or what brings us here today: your fertility journey.

No two fertility journeys will ever be the same. Maybe you have dreamt about becoming a parent your whole life. Maybe you never considered being a parent until that one person came into your life and made you rethink everything you thought you wanted or needed. Maybe you entered this journey unexpectedly.

I always knew I wanted to be a mother, but there was never a timeline or a rush to jump into that stage of my life . . . until there was. I thought getting pregnant was easy. I didn't see the struggles that people faced behind closed doors until I was the one behind the door. Our fertility journey was one of not *not* trying. We spent several years enjoying our marriage with the hopes that one day we would wake up to a surprise that our family was growing. After several years of wondering why I hadn't conceived yet, I was suddenly faced with questions of "*Can* we conceive? Is pregnancy even in the cards for us?"

In 2019, I was diagnosed with polycystic ovary syndrome, a hormone imbalance better known as PCOS. There was a laundry list of symptoms that I suffered from with the biggest being an irregular menstrual cycle or a lack thereof. This diagnosis became a major factor in our fertility journey and changed our approach to how we navigated the path to growing our family. As we both started researching different approaches to tackle the PCOS diagnosis, we found that food played a crucial role in managing symptoms and improving our chances of conceiving. Together with Tom's love for cooking and passion for serving others and my dedication to improving my health naturally, we set off on a journey to use food as medicine to support our fertility and overall well-being.

In 2022, that once "closed door" that we struggled behind became a window that we opened to the world when Tom and I published our first book, *Meals She Eats*. A cross between a cookbook and lifestyle book, *Meals She Eats* bridges the gap between research and personal experience, offering everything you need to know to naturally manage your diagnosis during each phase of your menstrual cycle. Through the tools of diet, exercise, and lifestyle changes, this book was created to help women who are in the same position as me get in tune with their bodies and overcome what they once thought were irreversible symptoms. It was created as not only a guide, but as the testimony of hope that we wish had existed after first receiving my diagnosis.

RACHAEL FINDS OUT SHE'S PREGNANT

RACHAEL: You will never forget the moment you find out you're pregnant for the first time. In a single instant, the trajectory of your whole life changes. You are instantly overwhelmed with emotions, both positive and negative, because, as exciting as it is, there is also a lot of unknown. It is a moment that will forever change you as a human being.

In the fall of 2021, I was working as a reserve flight attendant based in Charlotte, North Carolina, which meant I didn't hold a particular flying schedule, so my job was to be available when needed. If I was assigned to a flight, I was given a two-hour notice to get to the airport. Because we lived in Raleigh, North Carolina, I would commute into Charlotte for the day or a span of days. My aunt lived in town, so I was fortunate at the time to be able to stay at her place and avoid having to rent a hotel room for the day or sit at the airport where I would hang out until the airline called.

Sitting and waiting at my aunt's house, I had a lot of time to kill. It was not my intention to take a pregnancy test that day. Actually, I had what I thought was spotting with my period a few days prior, so I disregarded any notion that I was pregnant. That was until my friend Lauren educated me on implantation bleeding, which is a very normal thing that happens about 2 weeks after conception. There is so much *you don't know until you are pregnant*, and this was one of those things. Now, questioning myself and willing to do anything to pass the time until I got called to work a flight, I bought a pregnancy test, some tampons, and sour candy, in case I needed a pick-me-up from the disappointment of another negative test.

I ate the sour candy, not because I was disappointed, but because I was in disbelief that there were two pink lines on the pregnancy test I just took. I looked at the test, looked at myself in the mirror, and repeated the words "I don't believe it" more times than I could count. I sat on the toilet, held my belly, and cried. I cried and laughed; I cried and smiled; and then I stopped crying, picked up the test to triple check it, and dropped it again in disbelief. I just couldn't believe it was real. I had wanted this so badly I couldn't comprehend that it was actually happening. I stared at the test again and again and again and again.

Everyone experiences and registers this moment differently. Because Tom wasn't with me when I found out, I wanted to do something special for him. When we first started dating, we ate at a restaurant where you could doodle on the tablecloths. I had written "Rachael Sullivan" to see what my first name would look like with his last name added to it and then Tom responded by writing "Will you be?" and drew an arrow to my new name. I jokingly said yes and held onto that tablecloth as a memento of our relationship.

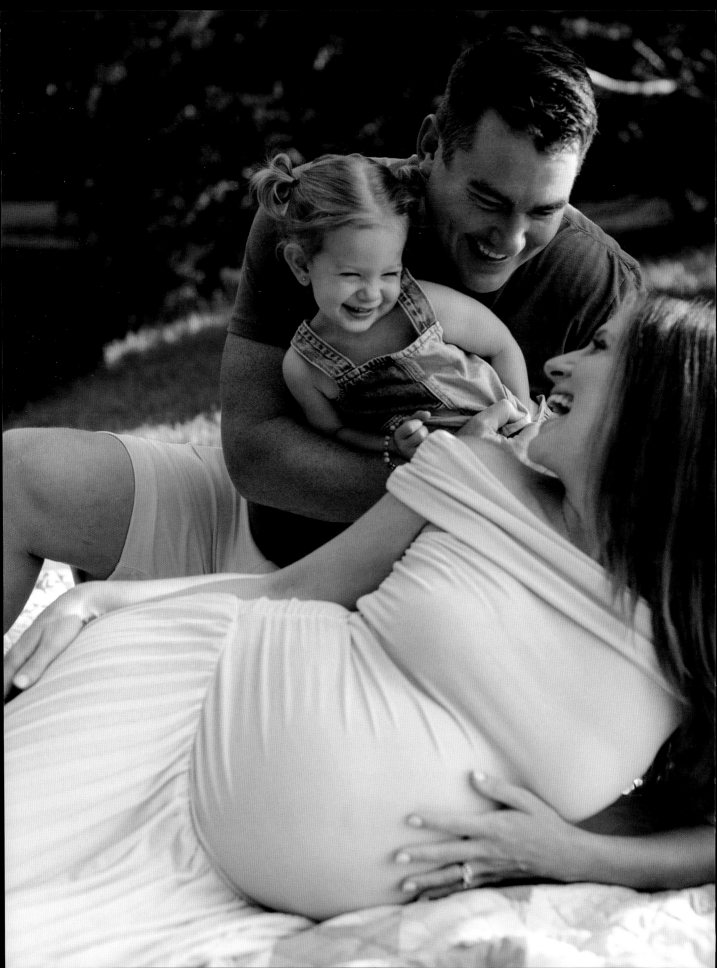

Tom also found significance in that tablecloth, because on the day he proposed, he used a photo of me sitting at that restaurant table with a note that read, "Do you remember 1,330 days ago when you joked about what your name would look like if this worked out?" In that moment, I was thankful I held onto that tablecloth because not only would I gift it to him the morning of our wedding, but years later, I would use it to tell him we were having a baby. It was the perfect artwork to hang in a baby's nursery after all. . .

TOM: Rachael was returning from a work trip just in time to help me host a cooking class for a bachelorette party. I don't remember a ton of the details from the event, but I remember we had a lot of fun, the food tasted great, and the exhaustion I felt after it was over was real. The plan was to collapse onto the couch for the rest of the afternoon and unwind. Little did I know, Rachael had other plans, and I was about to hear the most emotional and life-changing news of my life.

Rach entered the room, handing me something I immediately recognized: a framed tablecloth from one of our first dates. This tablecloth had become a cherished piece of our history together, and Rachael had often mentioned how she wanted it to hang in a nursery one day. As I had done in the past, I chuckled and replied, "We need a baby first." But today, her smile was different, and as she pulled out a pregnancy test and became emotional, my mind and heart went into overdrive.

A whirlwind of thoughts flooded me. I remembered she had mentioned spotting before her trip, leaving us both feeling defeated, so much so that I had scheduled a doctor's appointment to see if I could even have children. So when I saw the positive result, my first reaction was denial. I couldn't believe it—was she joking? Then came the avalanche of questions: Can we afford this? Will Rachael and I be able to handle it? Do we need to move? Will I be a good dad? Am I ready for this? In just a few moments, I cycled through what felt like a hundred different emotions, but looking into Rachael's eyes, everything became clear. My heart swelled with an overwhelming sense of joy and calm. It's a feeling I will never ever forget.

PREGNANCY TWO: ROSIE

RACHAEL: For almost 2 years, I thought about how I would tell Tom the exciting news if we ever got the chance to be pregnant again. I thought I would write him a letter from the baby saying that he or she was the size of a poppy seed and put a jar of poppy seed seasoning in a box for him to open, but that fairy tale I had in my head wasn't how the story unfolded. This time, pregnancy hit us when we least expected it and would be something we needed to navigate together with strength, love, and resilience.

It happened again . . . the implantation bleeding. This time, I knew deep down I was pregnant, but I was scared to find out. In October of 2023, Tom's mother, Lenore, was diagnosed with stage IV (four) lung cancer that had metastasized to her brain. We had spent 2 months driving back and forth from Raleigh to Chicago to help take care of her, and let's just say intimacy was not at the forefront of our relationship then. For almost 10 days, I knew I was pregnant, but I didn't want the confirmation because I was scared. I wasn't ready to add another variable to the mix. I felt as though I was the rock holding our family together, and I couldn't crack. This wasn't how I pictured entering a second pregnancy. I wanted to be selfish and celebrate, and I felt that I wasn't allowed to experience any of those emotions. How could I expect my husband or myself to feel happiness when his mother was battling for her life one day at a time. I couldn't comprehend the balance of grief and joy . . . it's still something I struggle with to this day.

Together at the Viceroy Hotel in downtown Chicago, Tom and I stood in the bathroom and took the pregnancy test together. For the first time in a long time, we were alone. We had spent the prior evening hosting a brand event in the city, and my parents were watching our daughter, Sutton, for the evening. We usually stayed at Tom's childhood home, alternating shifts with his siblings as caregivers for Lenore, but she was in the hospital being monitored after an episode, so there was no rush to go home. This privacy felt rare. With everything we had going on, we barely had a moment to ourselves. I knew then, if there was actually a chance that I was pregnant, this was the appropriate time to find out.

TOM: Before Rachael took the test, we talked about the stress we were under. I have to admit, the idea of it being positive scared the hell out of me. How could I possibly balance taking care of my mom, who lived 12 hours away and whose condition was deteriorating rapidly, while also being there for Rachael, Sutton, and now potentially another baby? I was scared, emotional, and overwhelmed. We knew we wanted more children, but with my mom's health in such a shaky state, it felt like all we could manage was getting through each day as it came.

RACHAEL: I don't think there was any part of Tom that actually thought it would be positive. We flipped over the test and both just stood in disbelief. The moment of disbelief never changes, but the type of disbelief does. At first, I wasn't consumed by all those emotions I had felt when finding out about my first pregnancy: the anticipation to become a mother, the joy, the excitement. Instead, I was consumed with fear and sadness. I felt that we had too much going on and that I wouldn't be able to take care of myself, let alone this baby.

TOM: When I saw the positive result, I was overcome with fear, uncertainty, and a sense of being completely overwhelmed. I wasn't immediately filled with the joy and excitement I felt during our first pregnancy. I felt like I was already falling short keeping up with my mom's situation, and now to think about everything a new pregnancy and eventually a new baby would bring was mentally draining. It was a strange, almost surreal moment—joy mixed with a profound sense of guilt and anxiety. Once the moment settled and some deep breaths were taken, that positive pregnancy test pulled from inside myself strength, courage, and even energy that I didn't know I had. In that moment, something shifted, and I felt ready—ready to be there for my wife, for Sutton, for our growing baby, for my mom, and for whatever else life would bring our way.

RACHAEL: I was never more thankful to have my husband by my side. He pulled me into his chest and held me. He asked about my fears. He reassured me that this was exciting news and that we would be able to get through this together. When I felt I couldn't breathe, he coached me through every breath. He was and still is my saving grace.

After being diagnosed with stage IV lung cancer in October of 2023, Tom's mom, Lenore Sullivan, passed away peacefully, surrounded by love on December 29, 2023, joining Tom's dad in their eternal home. Her one goal was to make it to Christmas, which she celebrated by having donuts for breakfast with all her kids and grandkids. Although Lenore never met Rosie, Tom and Rachael believe their souls met in passing to their final destinations.

After Lenore passed away, Rosie became the light in all our sadness. She was the motivation that pushed us to keep going, a reminder that even in the midst of grief, there was still hope and joy. Like a fragile bud pushing through the cold, hard ground, a symbol of life continuing even in the shadow of death, Rosie taught us both the depth of resilience and love.

HOW THIS BOOK CAME TO FRUITION

As my body grew babies from scratch, I found that one of the most exciting ways to provide updates was comparing our baby's growth to food. It's actually one of the most commonly asked questions: "What is my unborn baby's size this week?" I'm not sure why we think it's fun comparing our fetuses to fruit, but it is. The book you hold today is a symbol of how we celebrated our pregnancy on a weekly basis. Food had a key role in our fertility journey, and it extended into how we celebrated the weekly milestones of our pregnancy.

How did this all come to fruition you ask? When week 12 rolled around and our baby was the size of a fig, Tom ran out to our neighbor's fig tree that was in full bloom and picked some figs to show me the comparison. We took a picture of the fig next to my stomach as a keepsake, and then Tom had the idea to make some Arugula & Fig Pizza for lunch as a celebratory meal to honor this growth. As he was getting ready to dish up the pizza, I pulled out my camera and asked him, "Honey, what do we got?" From that week forward, we spent our Sundays in the kitchen making fun recipes that celebrated the baby's growth and shared our creations with the world. Whether it was Apple Nachos for week 15 or Roasted Butternut Squash Soup for week 35, we made a conscious effort to spend time each week reflecting on our journey.

Our hope for this book is that you embrace it as both a guide and a companion through the extraordinary journey of pregnancy. In doing so, we hope to provide support, nutritional guidance, and a way for you to consciously connect with your baby throughout the entire pregnancy process.

The book is broken down by each week of your pregnancy and divided into the three trimesters. Each week, we compare your baby's growth to the size of a fruit or vegetable, offering a fun and relatable way to visualize your baby's development. To accompany these milestones, we provide at least three recipes each week, ranging from mocktails and snacks to breakfast, lunch, dinner, and even dessert. You can cook one recipe, try them all, or save them for later—this is your journey, and it's all about flexibility and choice . . . and in my case, also cravings and aversions!

Every recipe is crafted with real, wholesome ingredients and is both gluten-free and dairy-free, building on the principles from our *New York Times* bestselling book, *Meals She Eats*. The variety and adaptability of our recipes allow you to tailor them to your tastes, cravings, or dietary needs, making each chapter a new opportunity for discovery and joy in your unique pregnancy experience. These dishes are designed not only to taste amazing, but also to aid in the nutrition needed to support both you and your growing baby, nourishing your body while celebrating the beautiful changes it undergoes.

Throughout the book, we also share personal stories that capture the unique experiences of pregnancy, offering emotional support and connection. We encourage you to explore each chapter not just as a guide, but as a journey of discovery and joy in your unique pregnancy experience. Dive into the stories, savor the recipes, and take a moment to reflect on how each week's development and nourishment parallels your own growth as a parent. Experiment with new ingredients, adapt the recipes to suit your cravings, and create your own rituals around these weekly milestones. Let each meal become a celebration and a chance to connect more deeply with your body, your baby, and the journey unfolding before you.

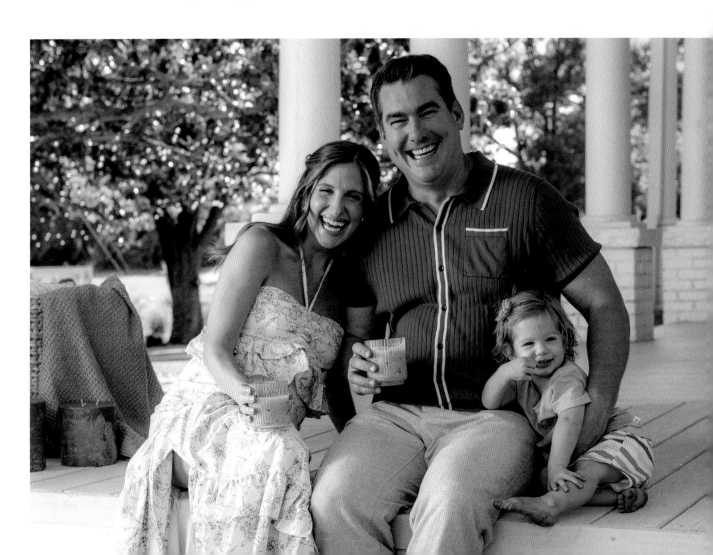

SIZE CHART

— week 8 —

blueberry

— week 9 —

raspberry

— week 10 —

cherry

— week 11 —

fig

— week 12 —

lime

— week 13 —

peach

— week 14 —

pear

— week 15 —

apple

— week 16 —

avocado

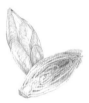

— week 17 —

endive

— week 18 —

pomegranate

— week 19 —

mango

— week 20 —

dragon fruit

— week 21 —

sweet potato

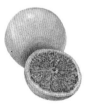

— week 22 —

grapefruit

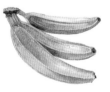

— week 23 —

banana

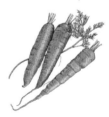

— week 24 —

carrots

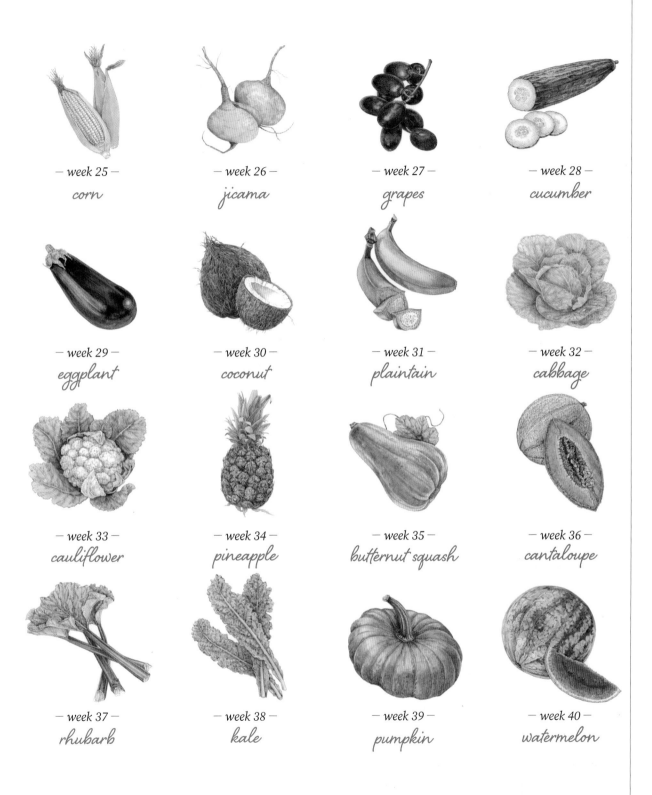

— week 25 —
corn

— week 26 —
jicama

— week 27 —
grapes

— week 28 —
cucumber

— week 29 —
eggplant

— week 30 —
coconut

— week 31 —
plaintain

— week 32 —
cabbage

— week 33 —
cauliflower

— week 34 —
pineapple

— week 35 —
butternut squash

— week 36 —
cantaloupe

— week 37 —
rhubarb

— week 38 —
kale

— week 39 —
pumpkin

— week 40 —
watermelon

WHAT SIZE IS YOUR BABY THIS WEEK?

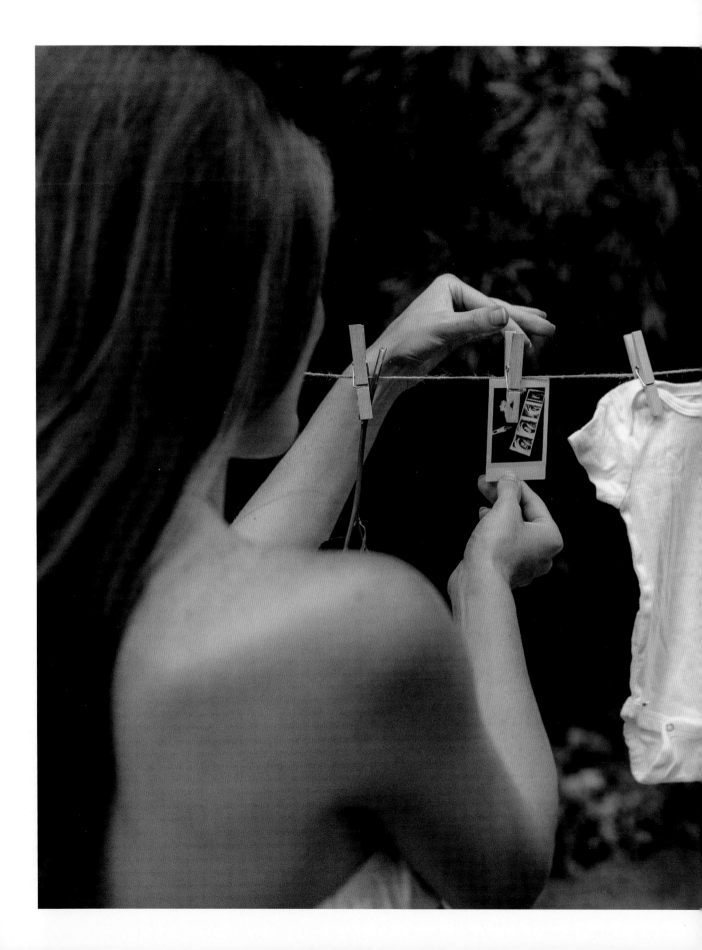

FIRST
TRIMESTER

*T*here is something so wonderful about the first trimester. The creation of life, and the days, if not weeks, in which you (and perhaps your partner) are the only one who knows about this little secret, this beautiful miracle of life. Over the course of these 12 weeks, your body is undergoing significant changes and will take on a transformation like never before, shifting not only your physical appearance, but your mental and emotional state too. While some symptoms may be what you anticipate, others might come as a surprise . . . like the way your body odor changes and you don't even recognize your own smell anymore. Expect the unexpected, and remember that each person's pregnancy experience is unique.

FIRST TRIMESTER MILESTONES

- Your little one's heart will begin to beat. If you remember to record this moment, it's a sound bite that you will cherish for the rest of time.

- Facial features will begin to form and those buds for arms and legs you see at the 8-week ultrasound appointment will start to develop. We always said the babies looked like little jelly beans at this stage.

- Your baby's organ's will develop and begin to function. Take a moment to think about the fact that you have two hearts (or more for multiple babies!) working inside of you. Never forget how incredible your body is.

- Fingernails and toenails will start to form. (Beware: Some babies, including mine, come out with claws!)

SYMPTOMS YOU MAY EXPERIENCE

- Breast tenderness and changes (Say hello to your new areolas, because they aren't going anywhere for a while.)
- Fatigue (Pregnancy fatigue is way worse than postpartum fatigue, and I stand by that.)
- Nausea and vomiting
- Heartburn and indigestion (The wives tale says your baby will have lots of hair if you experience these, but Rosie debunked this one.)
- Constipation (Invest in a good laxative.)

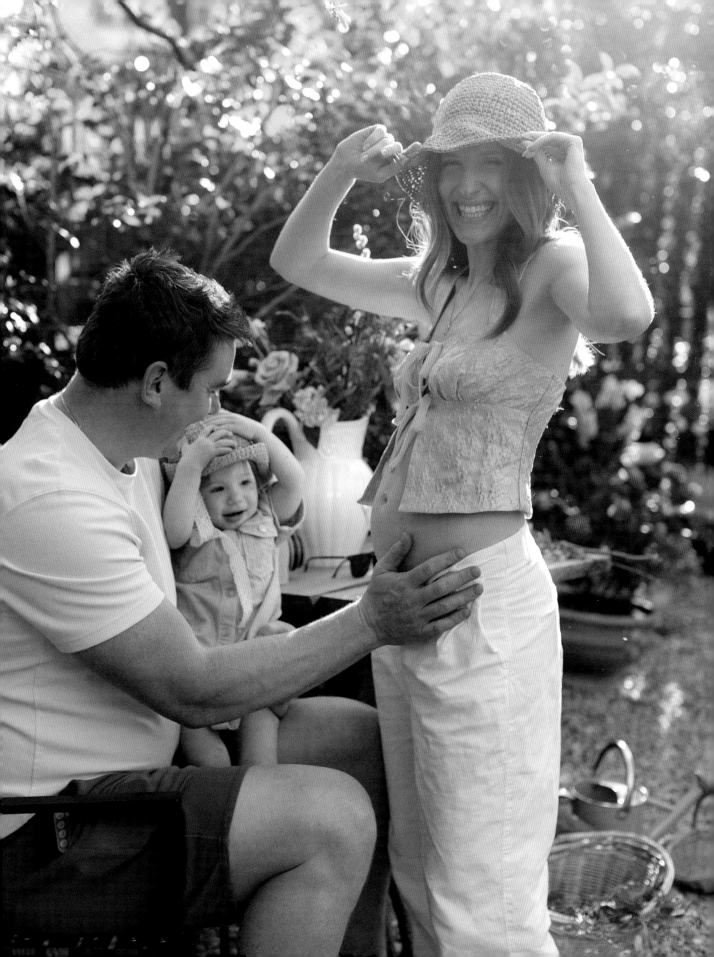

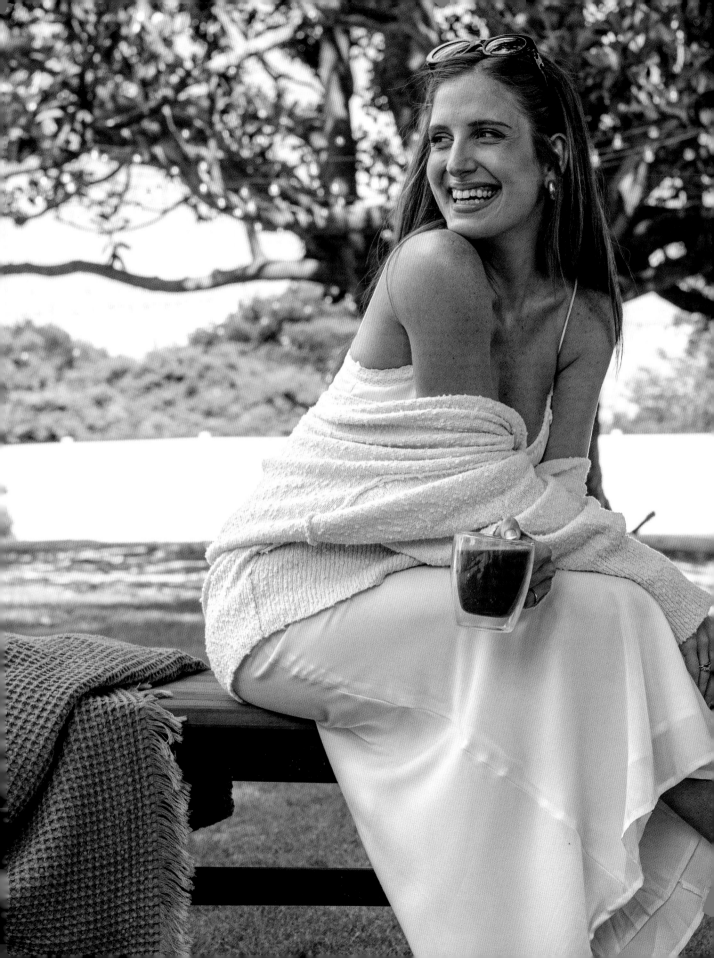

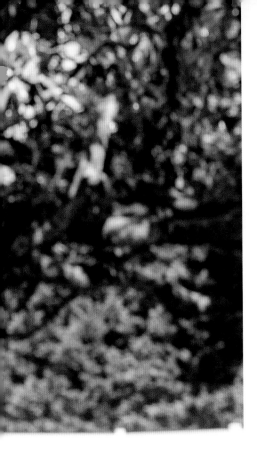

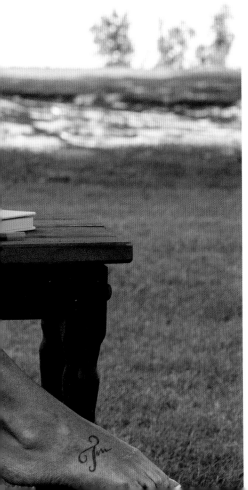

PREPARING FOR THIS SEASON

Embrace the journey with confidence. Whether you're in survival mode fitting in all the naps needed or you feel few to no symptoms, keep expectations to a minimum and know that your pregnancy will never have the same blueprint as somebody else's. The range of emotions that your hormones can bring about may have you hysterically laughing one minute and sobbing the next. Just know your feelings are valid and everything you're experiencing is temporary. What we can all relate to is taking the first trimester one day at a time, however that looks to you.

One of my favorite things at this stage is buying a journal to document not only your cherished memories, but also the challenges and hardships you face along the way. There will be plenty to document! Simmer in those moments of attending your first prenatal visits and seeing your baby during the ultrasound. Then, prepare for one of the most exciting things you get to do, deciding when and how you want to share the news with your loved ones and the world.

— week 8 —

BLUEBERRY SKILLET PANCAKE

Tom: Because every day should start with breakfast, let's begin with a classic staple: blueberry pancakes. But we're making it special by using my favorite kitchen tool, the cast-iron skillet. As my father-in-law often says, "You use that thing for everything—even the things you're not supposed to use it for!" And he's right—there's nothing it can't handle. If you're not a regular cast-iron user, grab yours and dust it off or treat yourself to a new one. This workhorse lasts forever. Cook up this blueberry pancake and watch as the edges crisp to perfection and the blueberries pop, releasing their sweet flavor to satisfy your cravings and kick off this celebration.

SERVINGS: 8	PREP TIME: 10 MINUTES	TOTAL TIME: 35 MINUTES

3 tablespoons avocado oil, divided
1 very ripe banana, mashed
1 cup almond milk
½ teaspoon vanilla extract
1 large egg
1½ cups almond flour
2 teaspoons baking powder
1 cup fresh blueberries

SERVING OPTIONS
Maple syrup
Fresh blueberries
Sliced banana

1 Preheat the oven to 425°F (220°C) and lightly oil an ovenproof 12-inch skillet with 1 tablespoon of avocado oil, making sure to coat the sides.

2 In a large bowl, combine the mashed banana, almond milk, remaining 2 tablespoons avocado oil, vanilla extract, and egg. Whisk until smooth.

3 Add the almond flour and baking powder to the wet ingredients. Whisk until the batter is well combined and smooth.

4 Gently fold the blueberries into the batter, being careful not to overmix.

5 Pour the batter into the prepared skillet. Tap the skillet on the counter to ensure the batter is evenly distributed.

6 Bake for about 20 minutes or until a toothpick inserted into the center of the pancake comes out clean.

7 Allow the pancake to cool for a minute or two, then cut into 8 slices for serving.

8 Serve with maple syrup, additional fresh blueberries, and sliced bananas, if desired.

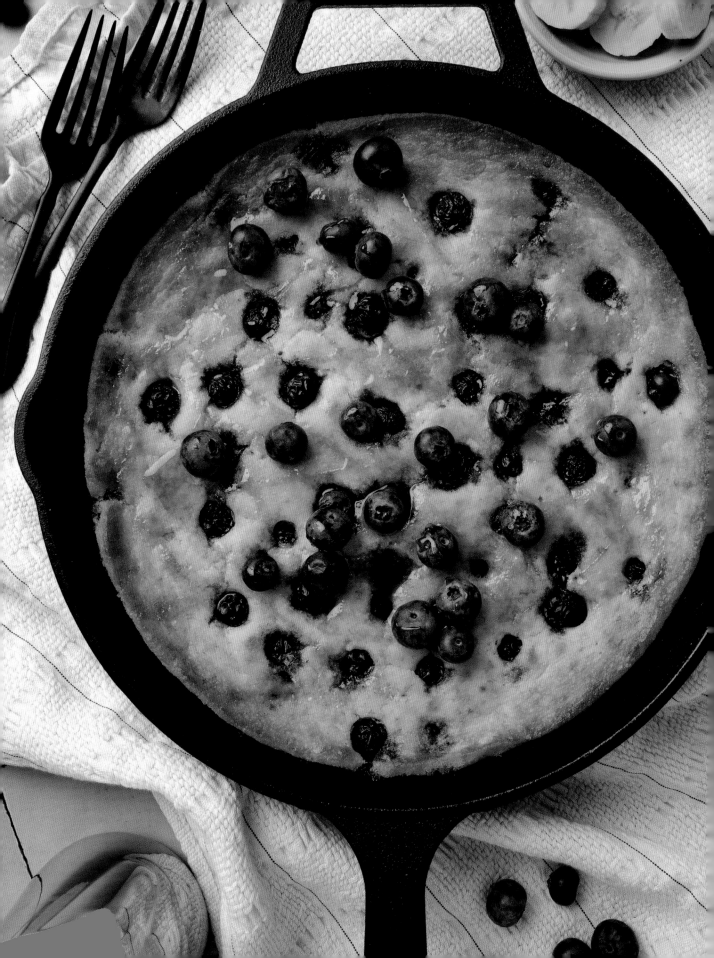

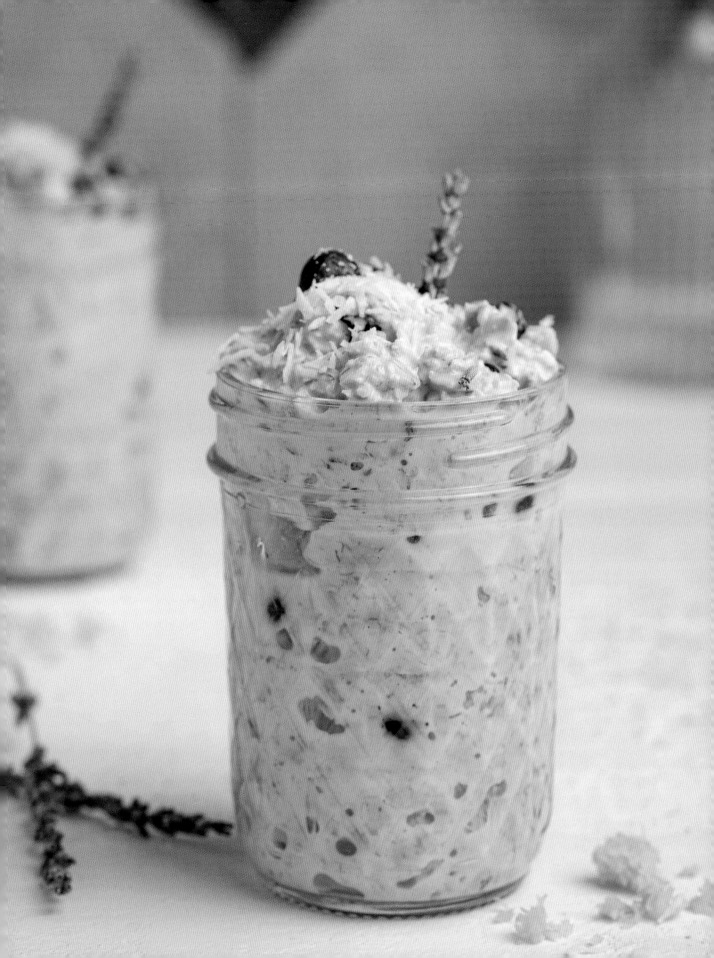

LEMON, BLUEBERRY & LAVENDER OVERNIGHT OATS

Rachael: Not only physical fatigue but decision fatigue is so real when it comes to pregnancy. Overnight oats take the thought process out of *what should I eat this morning* because you already did the prep work the night before. This is a fun dish that not only tastes good but is high in fiber and rich in nutrients for you and baby.

SERVINGS: 2	PREP TIME: 10 MINUTES	TOTAL TIME: 10 MINUTES, PLUS 4 HOURS OR OVERNIGHT TO CHILL

1 cup gluten-free rolled oats

1 cup unsweetened almond milk or milk of choice

1 tablespoon honey or maple syrup (adjust to taste)

1 tablespoon fresh lemon juice

1 teaspoon lemon zest

½ teaspoon dried culinary-grade lavender

Pinch of salt

⅓ cup fresh blueberries

SERVING OPTIONS

Fresh blueberries

Lemon wedges

Toasted coconut flakes

Slivered almonds

1 In a medium bowl, combine the rolled oats, almond milk, honey, lemon juice, lemon zest, dried lavender, and a pinch of salt. Stir well to combine all the ingredients evenly.

2 Gently fold in the blueberries until evenly distributed throughout the mixture.

3 Cover the bowl or jar with plastic wrap or a lid and refrigerate for 4 hours or overnight to allow the oats to soften and absorb the liquid.

4 Once the oats have chilled and thickened, give them a stir. If desired, you can add a splash of additional almond milk to adjust the consistency.

5 Divide the overnight oats into serving bowls or jars.

6 Garnish with additional fresh blueberries, lemon wedges, toasted coconut flakes, and slivered almonds, if desired.

— week 8 —

BLUEBERRY & CHIPOTLE CHICKEN

Tom: The day I found out how amazing chipotle peppers in adobo sauce were, I basically made it one of my life's missions to find out how many ways I can use them in recipes. This dish certainly did not disappoint. The sweetness of the blueberries perfectly balances the smoky, spicy kick of chipotle, creating an amazing combination. Sweet and savory is a hard combo to beat, and I love that the simmer time allows the flavors to come together while giving you time to prep sides or simply relax.

SERVINGS: 4	PREP TIME: 10 MINUTES	TOTAL TIME: 30 MINUTES

4 boneless, skinless chicken breasts
Salt and pepper, to taste
1 tablespoon olive oil

FOR THE SAUCE
1 (7-ounce/198g) can chipotle peppers in adobo sauce
1 cup frozen blueberries, thawed
2 garlic cloves, minced
1 tablespoon apple cider vinegar
1 tablespoon honey or maple syrup
1 tablespoon coconut aminos or gluten-free soy sauce
1 teaspoon ground cumin
½ teaspoon smoked paprika

SERVING OPTIONS
Fresh cilantro, chopped
Lime wedges
Steamed vegetables
Quinoa
Rice

1 Season the chicken breasts with salt and pepper on both sides.

2 **Prepare the sauce.** To a blender or food processor, add 2 chipotle peppers (reserve remaining peppers and sauce for a future use) and all the remaining sauce ingredients and then blend until smooth. Taste and add more adobo sauce or honey, as desired.

3 Heat the olive oil in a large skillet over medium-high heat. Once hot, add the seasoned chicken breasts to the skillet and sear for 2 to 3 minutes on each side, until golden brown.

4 Reduce the heat to medium-low and pour the blueberry-chipotle sauce over the chicken in the skillet, ensuring that the chicken is coated evenly with the sauce.

5 Allow the chicken to simmer in the sauce for 10 to 15 minutes. Flip the chicken occasionally, spooning the sauce over the top to ensure it's well-coated and infused with flavor.

6 Once the chicken is cooked through and reaches an internal temperature of 165°F (74°C), remove the skillet from the heat.

7 Garnish the chicken with chopped fresh cilantro, if desired.

8 Serve with lime wedges, along with your favorite side dish, such as steamed vegetables, quinoa, or rice, if desired.

Note *For lunch, we love to serve this as a bowl over brown rice or arugula with roasted sweet potato, roasted broccoli, chickpeas, fresh avocado, pumpkin seeds, and pickled red onion.*

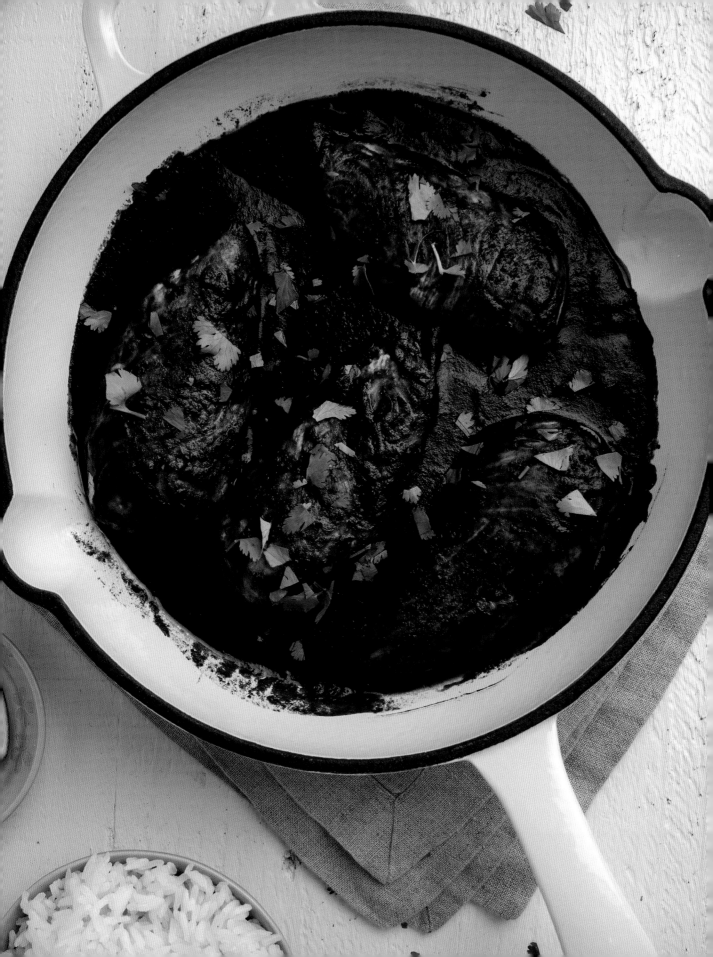

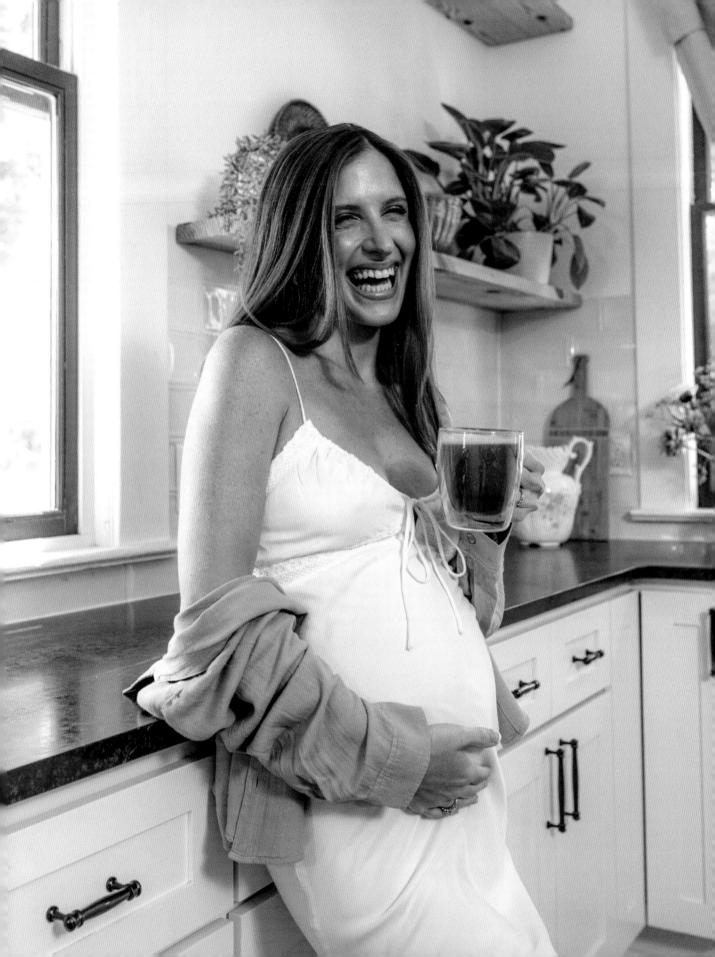

RASPBERRY GINGER TEA

Rachael: Raspberry-leaf tea is something you might become very familiar with toward the end of your pregnancy when you're ready for the baby's arrival. It has been known to aid labor and postpartum recovery with its magical side effects for a quicker, easier delivery. This recipe incorporates ginger and honey for added health benefits and will be a page to bookmark for later, when you are in the final stretch, curb-walking, and ready for the baby to come out.

SERVINGS: 2–3	**PREP TIME:** 10 MINUTES	**TOTAL TIME:** 15 MINUTES

2 cups almond milk
2 raspberry-leaf tea bags
1 cup fresh raspberries, rinsed
Fresh ginger, 1-inch (2.5cm) piece, peeled and thinly sliced
½ teaspoon vanilla extract
Pinch of sea salt
1 tablespoon honey, or to taste
Fresh mint leaves, optional, for garnish

1 In a small saucepan, bring the milk to a simmer over medium heat.

2 Once the milk comes to a simmer, turn off the heat and add the tea bags. Steep for 5 minutes.

3 While the tea is steeping, add the raspberries, ginger, vanilla extract, salt, and honey to a blender. After the steeping is finished, remove the tea bags from the milk tea and pour the it into the blender. Blend until smooth.

4 Pour the tea through a fine-mesh sieve or cheesecloth to remove the ginger and any raspberry seeds.

5 Pour the strained tea into mugs or teacups. Taste and add honey if you would like a sweeter tea. Garnish with fresh mint, if desired.

RASPBERRY DIJON CHICKEN

Tom: The cooking technique used in this recipe is one of my favorite ways to prepare a main protein. To me, it's the elevated sheet pan. Sheet pan recipes end up lacking texture and flavor, but starting them on the stovetop in a cast-iron or ovenproof pan and getting a good sear locks in the juices and adds great texture. Then just add your sauce and bake. In this case, the sauce is a raspberry Dijon that is versatile and tastes sweet, tangy, and savory. I would use this sauce on salmon or even as a marinade for flank steak.

SERVINGS: 4	**PREP TIME:** 5 MINUTES	**TOTAL TIME:** 35 MINUTES

4 boneless, skinless chicken breasts
Salt and pepper
1 tablespoon olive oil
½ cup chicken broth

FOR THE SAUCE
¼ cup raspberry preserves, no-sugar-added or naturally sweetened
2 tablespoons Dijon mustard
2 garlic cloves, minced
1 tablespoon apple cider vinegar
Salt and pepper, to taste

SERVING OPTIONS
Fresh raspberries
Chopped fresh parsley
Steamed vegetables
Quinoa
Cooked brown or basmati rice

1 Preheat the oven to 375°F (190°C).

2 Season the chicken breasts with salt and pepper on both sides.

3 In an ovenproof skillet, heat the olive oil over medium-high heat. Once hot, add the chicken breasts to the skillet and sear for 2 to 3 minutes on each side, until golden brown.

4 **Prepare the sauce.** In a small bowl, whisk together all the sauce ingredients until well combined.

5 Pour the sauce over the seared chicken breasts in the skillet. Gently pour the broth around the chicken.

6 Transfer the skillet to the preheated oven and bake for 20 to 25 minutes or until the chicken is cooked through and reaches an internal temperature of 165°F (74°C).

7 While baking, occasionally baste the chicken with the sauce in the skillet to keep it moist and flavorful.

8 Once the chicken is cooked through, remove the skillet from the oven. Allow 4 to 5 minutes to rest on a cutting board, cut chicken into slices, and garnish with a drizzle of the reserved sauce from the pan. Top with fresh raspberries and chopped parsley, if using.

9 Serve immediately along with your favorite side dish, such as steamed vegetables, quinoa, or rice, if desired.

Note This is a great protein for a salad. We love pairing it with spinach and arugula mix, walnuts, thinly sliced red onion, thinly sliced fresh basil, diced apples, goat cheese, and raspberry vinaigrette.

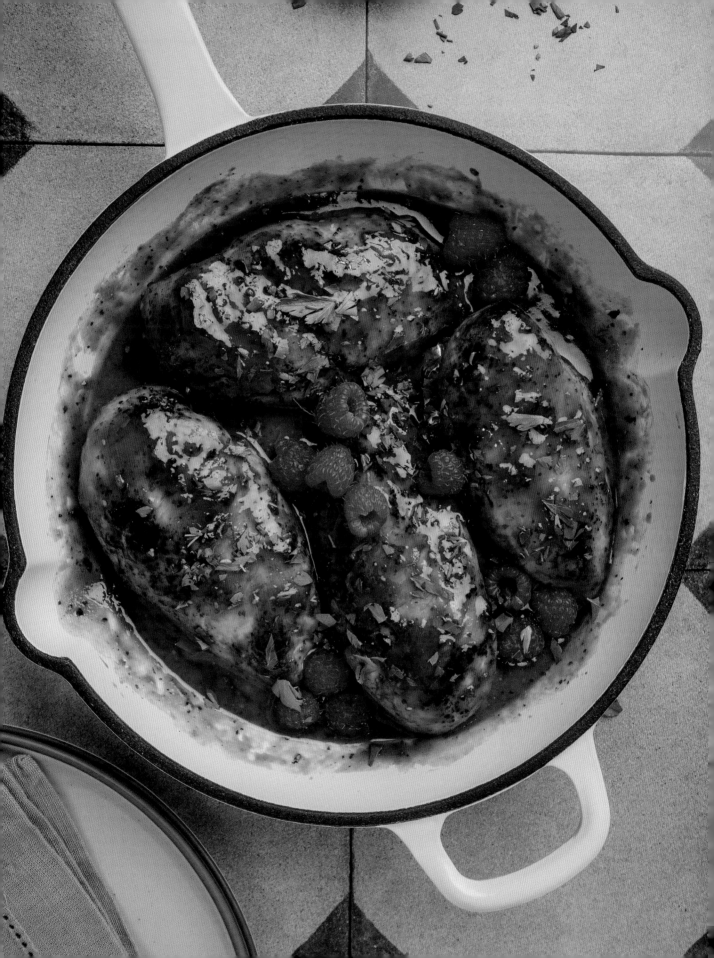

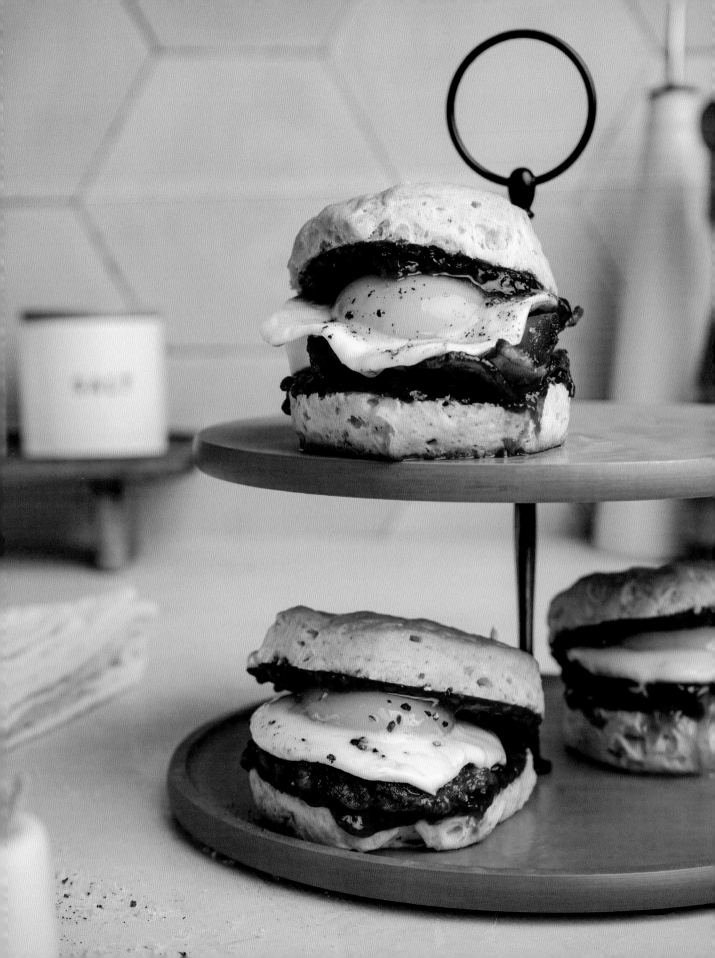

RASPBERRY MARMALADE BREAKFAST SLIDERS

Rachael: If you've never had jam on a breakfast slider, today is your lucky day. (That is unless you've been dealing with the typical morning sickness that comes with the first trimester, then my heart goes out to you.) I've found the best way to offset the onset of nausea is by eating every three hours, and sometimes, nothing sounds better than a sandwich. The combination of carbs, fat, and protein—and for me, a little touch of sweetness—always hit the spot.

SERVINGS: 2	PREP TIME: 10 MINUTES	TOTAL TIME: 35 MINUTES

2 cups fresh raspberries, rinsed
¼ cup water
¼ cup honey
Zest and juice of 1 lemon
4 strips of bacon or 2 breakfast sausage patties
2 large eggs
2 gluten-free biscuits, halved; or 4 gluten-free bread slices; or 2 small gluten-free rolls, halved
Salt and pepper, to taste
Dash of hot sauce, optional

1 Add the raspberries, water, and honey to a medium pot over medium heat. Allow to cook, stirring occasionally, until the raspberries start to burst.

2 Add the lemon zest and juice to the raspberries. Stir and cook for 10 to 12 minutes, until all berries have burst and the mixture becomes smooth and thick. Remove from the heat and set the marmalade aside.

3 Once the marmalade is done, preheat the oven to 325°F (165°C) and begin cooking the breakfast meat and eggs.

4 In a large skillet over medium heat, cook the bacon until cooked through, 7 to 8 minutes, flipping once.

5 Reduce the heat to medium and shift the bacon to one side of the skillet.

6 Add the eggs to the empty side of the skillet and cook to desired doneness, 3 minutes for sunny-side up.

7 While the eggs are cooking, place your bread in the preheated oven for 4 minutes to warm.

8 To assemble the sliders, spread a tablespoon of marmalade on the top and bottom piece of each biscuit. Place 2 slices of bacon (or 1 sausage patty) on the bottom piece of biscuit, followed by an egg and season with salt and pepper.

9 Add a dash of hot sauce over the eggs, if desired. Complete the sliders by placing the top pieces of biscuit over the eggs.

10 Store remaining marmalade inside an airtight container in the fridge for up to 3 weeks.

CHERRY VINAIGRETTE WEDGE SALAD

Rachael: This wedge salad is a super fun recipe because you get to learn the art of making croutons and vinaigrette from scratch. Both recipes are very easy, might I add, and you'll wonder why you never thought to attempt them sooner. As a member of the gluten-free society, I find a good crouton is imperative, and I have been known to hide a stash of these in my purse to enjoy with my salads at restaurants from time to time— pregnancy cravings be like that.

SERVINGS: 4	PREP TIME: 15 MINUTES	TOTAL TIME: 30 MINUTES

¼ cup pine nuts
1 large head iceberg lettuce, quartered into 4 wedges
½ cup pickled red onion
½ cup pitted and chopped fresh cherries or sweetened dried cherries
½ cup watermelon radish matchsticks

FOR THE CROUTONS
4 slices gluten-free bread
½ teaspoon smoked paprika
½ teaspoon garlic powder
Salt and pepper, to taste
1 tablespoon olive oil, to lightly coat the bread, more as needed

FOR THE BALSAMIC VINAIGRETTE
1 cup pitted fresh cherries
⅓ cup extra-virgin olive oil
⅓ cup apple cider vinegar
Pinch of salt

1 **Prepare the croutons.** Preheat the oven to 425°F (220°C). Cut the bread (preferably stale but fresh works as well) into cubes.

2 To a medium bowl, add the bread, paprika, garlic powder, salt, and pepper. Drizzle in the olive oil, and toss well to combine.

3 Spread the tossed croutons evenly on a baking sheet lined with parchment paper. Place the croutons into the preheated oven, and bake for 10 minutes before removing from the oven and flipping the squares. Add the pine nuts to the baking sheet alongside the flipped squares and bake for an additional 3 to 5 minutes. Remove and let cool.

4 **Prepare the vinaigrette.** Add all the vinaigrette ingredients to a blender, and blend on high until smooth. Check the flavor and add additional salt if desired.

5 Lay each lettuce wedge on a plate and top with red onion, cherries, and watermelon radish. Drizzle the vinaigrette over everything and then top with croutons and toasted pine nuts.

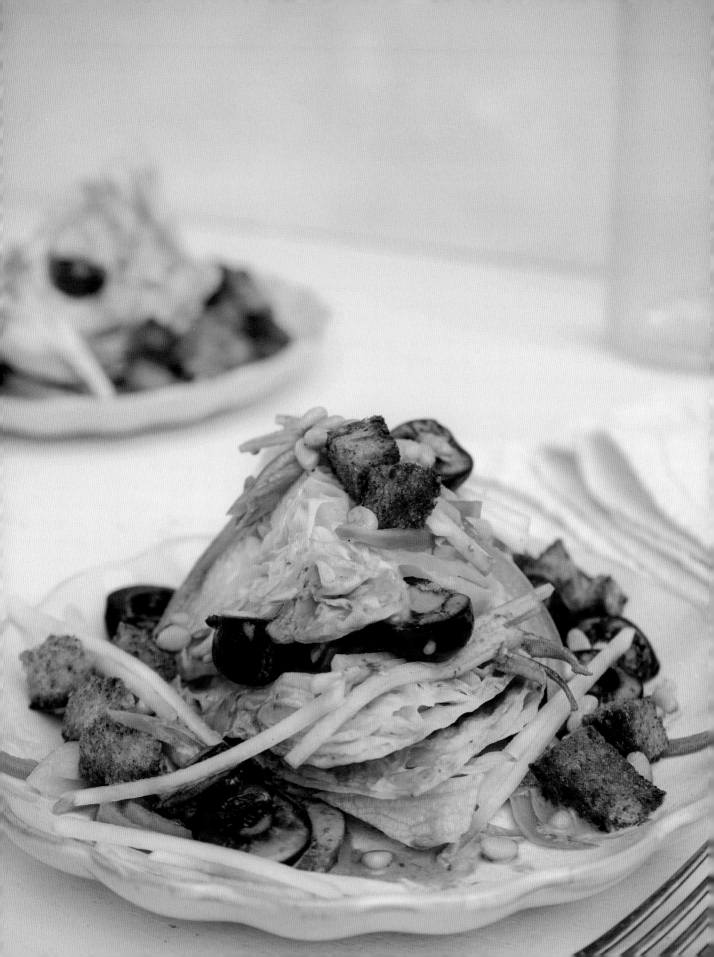

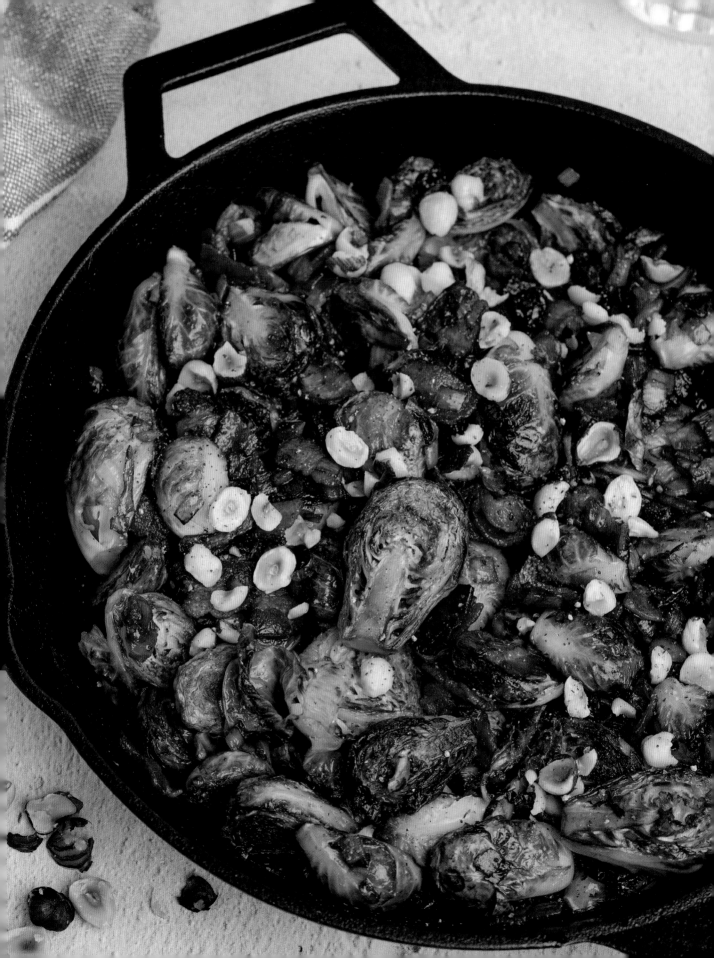

CHERRY-BALSAMIC BRUSSELS SPROUTS

Tom: I hated brussels sprouts growing up, and we only had them one way: frozen in a plastic bag, smothered in cheese, that you boiled to warm up. I don't think I ate a brussels sprout for 10 years once I left my parents' house. But then I rediscovered them and how versatile they can be. This is a sweet and salty side dish that will become a staple in your home, just like it has in ours.

SERVINGS: 2–4	PREP TIME: 10 MINUTES	TOTAL TIME: 40 MINUTES

1 pound (450g) brussels sprouts
½ pound (225g) thinly sliced bacon or cubed pancetta
Salt and pepper, to taste
1 shallot, diced
½ cup naturally sweetened dried cherries
1 tablespoon balsamic vinegar
Drizzle of balsamic glaze, optional
¼ cup chopped walnuts or hazelnuts, toasted

1 Bring a large pot filled with salted water to a boil over high heat.

2 Add the brussels sprouts to the boiling water and boil for 2 to 4 minutes until they turn bright green. Transfer to a paper towel and allow to cool.

3 In a large pan over medium heat, cook the bacon for 5 to 7 minutes, rendering the fat. Remove bacon with a slotted spoon. Discard most of the fat, leaving 1 to 2 tablespoons in the pan.

4 When cooled, trim the brussels sprouts and cut in half lengthwise.

5 Add the brussels sprouts, cut side down, to the pan, and season with salt and pepper. Cook undisturbed for 6 to 8 minutes until they brown and are caramelized on the bottom.

6 Add the cooked bacon, shallot, cherries, and balsamic vinegar to the pan. Season with additional salt and pepper and sauté for 4 minutes. Transfer to a platter or bowl for serving.

7 If desired, drizzle the brussels sprouts with balsamic glaze and toss gently to coat all the ingredients evenly. Top with toasted walnuts.

— week 10 —

CHERRY & ROSEMARY CHICKEN

Tom: I remember when we were creating this recipe, we tried all kinds of crazy and over-the-top things. For example, pickling different types of cherries or creating a cherry "cure" to dry-age the chicken. Then we made a simple recipe combining some of our favorite ingredients like rosemary, balsamic vinegar, honey, and onion. Add the serendipity of the baby being the size of a cherry and a home-run meal was created. Sometimes, sticking to what you know you already love is the best way to go!

SERVINGS: 2–3	**PREP TIME:** 10 MINUTES	**TOTAL TIME:** 50 MINUTES, PLUS 1 HOUR OR OVERNIGHT TO MARINATE

2 tablespoons cherry preserves

¼ cup balsamic vinegar

2 tablespoons honey

¼ cup plus 1 tablespoon olive oil, divided

Salt and pepper, to taste

4 to 6 bone-in, skin-on chicken thighs

3 sprigs fresh rosemary

½ sweet onion, sliced

1 cup cherries , fresh or frozen, pitted and halved

Cooked basmati or brown rice, for serving

1 In a small bowl, stir together the cherry preserves, balsamic vinegar, honey, ¼ cup olive oil, salt, and pepper. Pour the marinade into a large zipper-lock bag and add the chicken thighs. Seal and place in the fridge to marinate for at least 1 hour or overnight.

2 Preheat the oven to 425°F (220°C). Remove the chicken from the fridge and let sit for 15 minutes to come to room temperature.

3 Place a large cast-iron skillet or ovenproof pan over medium-high heat. Coat the pan with the remaining 1 tablespoon olive oil.

4 Once the oil is hot, place the chicken thighs into the skillet skin side down, reserving the marinade. You should hear it sizzle. Cook for 3 to 5 minutes. Flip the chicken skin side up. Nestle the rosemary, sweet onion slices, and cherries among the chicken thighs. Pour the reserved marinade into the skillet.

5 Transfer the skillet to the oven and cook for 12 to 18 minutes or until the internal temperature of the chicken reaches 165°F (74°C).

6 Remove the skillet from the oven and serve the chicken over rice. Remove the rosemary sprigs and drizzle the pan sauce over the chicken and rice.

Note *This recipe can also be prepared with skin-on salmon approximately 1½ pounds (680g), cooked the same way until the internal temperature 145°F (63°C).*

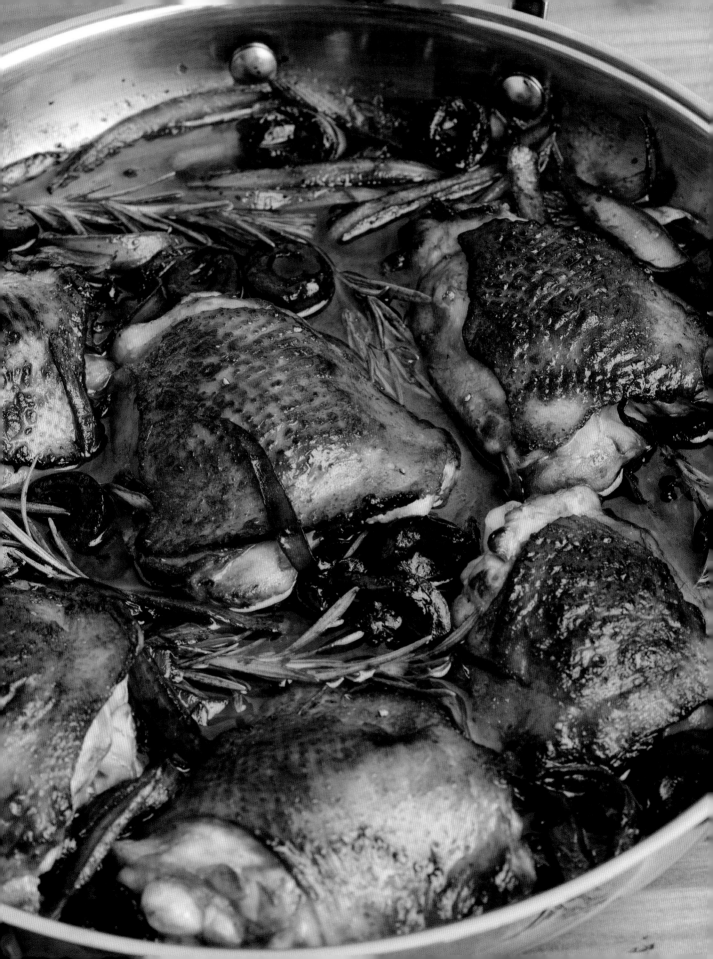

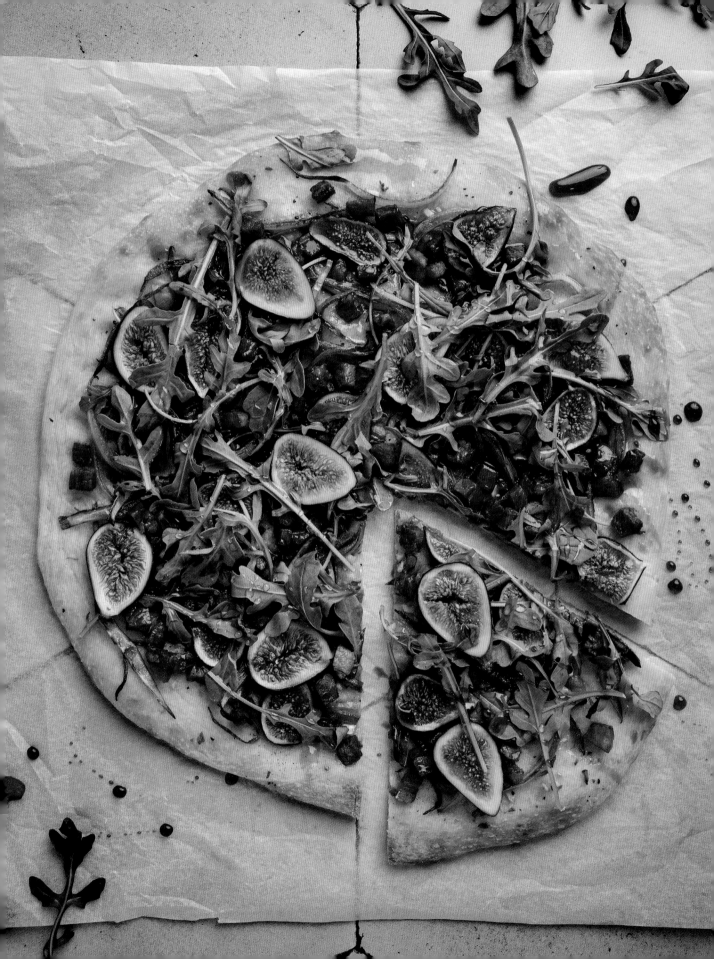

ARUGULA & FIG PIZZA

Rachael: Oh, this is the recipe that started it all, and my honey did not disappoint with this combination. A rustic touch of Italian flavors with a hot honey twist, this pizza might inspire a babymoon to Italy, and we will take full blame for that.

SERVINGS: 8	PREP TIME: 10 MINUTES	TOTAL TIME: 40 MINUTES

2 tablespoons coconut oil
½ white onion, thinly sliced
Pinch of salt
1 (12-inch/30cm) cauliflower pizza crust
1 tablespoon olive oil
2 garlic cloves, minced
Pinch of black pepper
1 tablespoon balsamic vinegar
5 ounces (142g) pancetta, finely diced
2–3 fresh figs, thinly sliced
1 cup arugula
Drizzle of balsamic glaze, optional
Drizzle of hot honey, optional

1 Preheat the oven to 425°F (220°C).

2 Heat the coconut oil in a medium pan over medium heat. Add the onion and a pinch of salt. Cook the onion until translucent, about 5 to 7 minutes.

3 Meanwhile, place the cauliflower crust on a pizza pan and evenly coat it with olive oil, garlic, and pepper. Set aside.

4 Once the onion slices are translucent, add the balsamic vinegar and cook for 2 to 3 minutes more, until slightly caramelized.

5 Spread the onion evenly over the prepared cauliflower crust.

6 In the pan the onion was removed from, cook the pancetta over medium heat for 5 to 7 minutes until some of the fat renders. Remove the pan from the heat and spread the pancetta evenly over the crust, discarding the fat.

7 Spread the sliced figs evenly over the onion and pancetta.

8 Bake the pizza for 12 to 17 minutes..

9 Remove the pizza from the oven and top with arugula, then drizzle with balsamic glaze and hot honey, if desired.

— week 11 —

FIG & WALNUT CORNBREAD

Rachael: I love food that looks and tastes beautiful, and this fig and walnut cornbread is just that. The rustic feel of the cast iron, the warmth of the cornbread itself, and the surprise element of figs when you flip the dish over has me in my cozy nesting feels. The dish looks like a piece of art that you almost feel guilty biting into, but not guilty enough that you don't.

SERVINGS: 8–10	PREP TIME: 10 MINUTES	TOTAL TIME: 30 MINUTES

2 cups cornmeal
1 teaspoon salt
½ teaspoon baking powder
½ teaspoon baking soda
2 large eggs
1½ cups almond milk
1 teaspoon lemon zest
2 tablespoons lemon juice
½ cup maple syrup
½ cup melted lard or oil of choice, divided
8 fresh figs, halved
1 cup chopped walnuts

1. Place a 10-inch (25cm) cast-iron skillet inside the oven and then preheat the oven to 425°F (220°C).

2. In a medium bowl, whisk together the cornmeal, salt, baking powder, and baking soda.

3. Once the dry ingredients are combined, add the eggs, almond milk, lemon zest, lemon juice, maple syrup, and ¼ cup of the melted lard to the bowl and stir to combine until a batter is formed.

4. Carefully remove the hot skillet from the preheated oven, leaving the oven on. Add the remaining ¼ cup of melted lard to the skillet and swirl the skillet around to coat all of the inside well.

5. Place the figs cut side down into the skillet and add the walnuts. Pour the batter over the top to cover the figs and walnuts. Carefully shake the skillet back and forth lightly to settle the batter.

6. Return the skillet to the oven and bake for 20 minutes. Check for doneness with a toothpick or paring knife by inserting into the center and if the toothpick pulls out clean and the cornbread slightly pulls away from the sides of pan, the cornbread is ready.

7. Remove from the oven and allow to cool slightly before slicing and serving.

Note *This recipe can also be made with dried figs. If using dried, soak the figs in hot water for 30 minutes before using.*

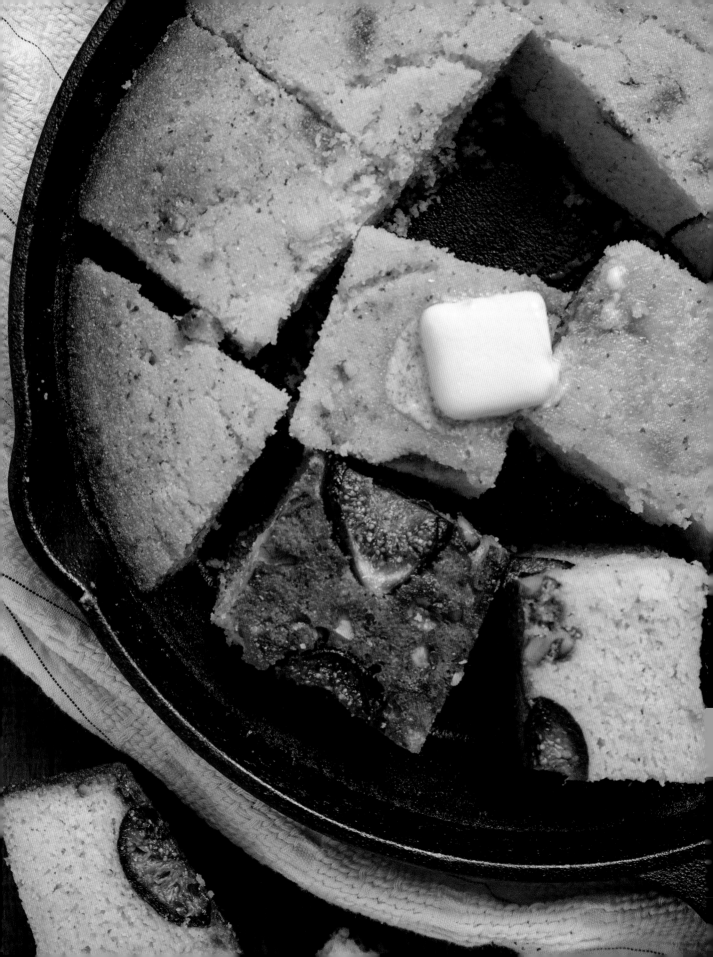

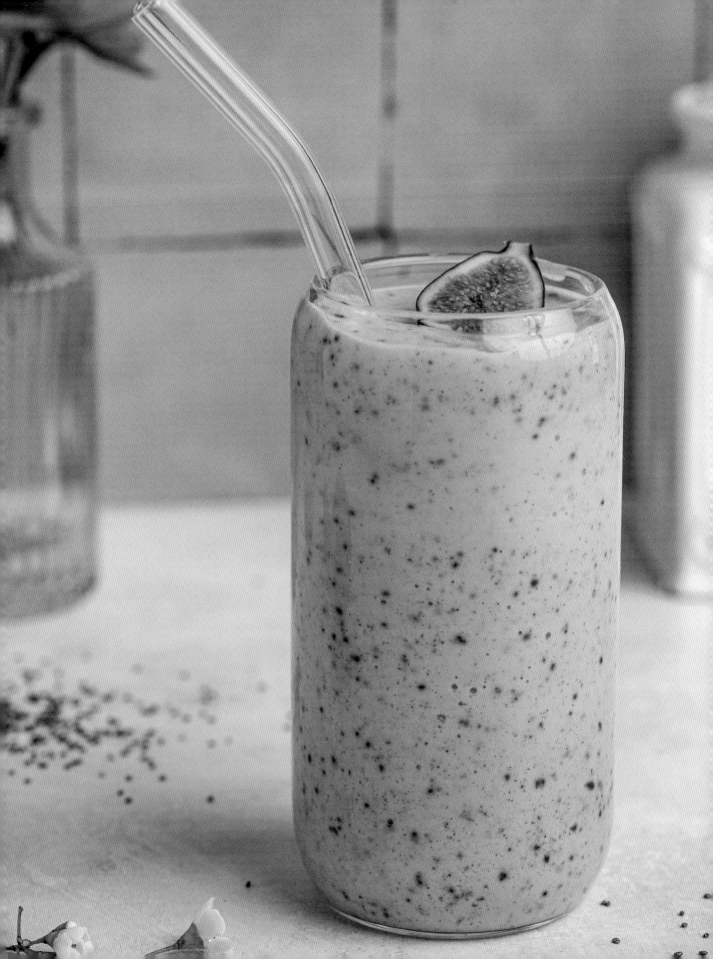

— week 11 —

FIG & BANANA SMOOTHIE

Rachael: I drank smoothies on repeat during the early stages of pregnancy when food sounded not so appetizing. At this point in your pregnancy, you might also be feeling the same way. If you have been craving something cold that you can sip on, then hopefully this fig and banana smoothie will be a refreshing addition to your week!

SERVINGS: 2	PREP TIME: 5 MINUTES	TOTAL TIME: 7–10 MINUTES

1 ripe banana

4 to 5 dried figs, stems removed and chopped

½ cup plain dairy-free or Greek yogurt

½ cup unsweetened almond milk or milk of your choice

1 tablespoon almond butter or cashew butter

½ teaspoon ground cinnamon

¼ teaspoon vanilla extract

1 tablespoon chia seeds or ground flaxseeds, optional

Ice cubes, optional

Drizzle of honey, optional

1 In a blender, combine banana, figs, yogurt, milk, almond butter, cinnamon, vanilla extract, and chia seeds, if using, and blend on high until smooth and creamy. If the smoothie is too thick, thin it out with additional almond milk or water. If the smoothie is too thin, add a few ice cubes and blend again until smooth to thicken it.

2 Taste the smoothie, and adjust the sweetness with a drizzle of honey if you prefer a sweeter flavor.

3 Pour the smoothie into glasses and serve immediately.

KEY LIME PIE OVERNIGHT OATS

Rachael: If your pregnancy cravings have started and you find yourself reaching for sweet treats already, then these key lime pie overnight oats will be sure to satisfy that dessert craving. Instead of giving you a sugar crash like donuts or cereal, oats will leave you feeling nourished for the rest of the day and—trust me—reserving your energy sources are crucial at this stage of pregnancy.

SERVINGS: 2	**PREP TIME:** 5 MINUTES	**TOTAL TIME:** 5 MINUTES, PLUS 4 HOURS OR OVERNIGHT TO CHILL

1 cup gluten-free rolled oats

1 cup unsweetened almond milk or milk of choice

Zest of 1 key lime or 1 small lime

2 tablespoons key lime juice or lime juice

2 tablespoons honey or maple syrup

½ teaspoon vanilla extract

2 tablespoons plain dairy-free or Greek yogurt

1 tablespoon chia seeds

Pinch of salt

1 tablespoon unsweetened shredded coconut, optional

Sliced key limes or lime wedges, optional, to garnish

1 In a medium mixing bowl, add the oats, almond milk, key lime zest, lime juice, honey, vanilla extract, yogurt, chia seeds, and salt, as well as the shredded coconut, if using. Stir well to combine.

2 Cover the bowl with plastic wrap or a lid, and refrigerate the mixture for 4 hours or overnight to allow the oats to soften and absorb the flavors.

3 Once the oats have chilled and thickened, stir them well. If the mixture is too thick, you can add a little more almond milk to reach desired consistency.

4 Divide the overnight oats into serving bowls or jars, garnish with sliced key limes or lime wedges, if desired, and serve.

Note   *You can adjust the sweetness of the overnight oats by using more or less honey or maple syrup, depending on your preferences.*

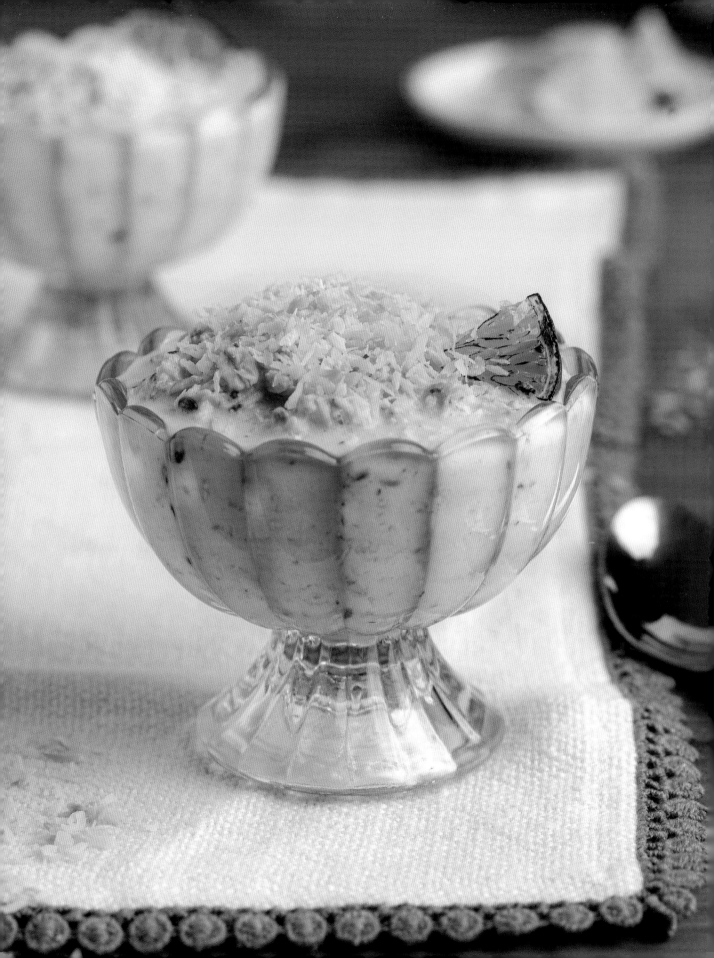

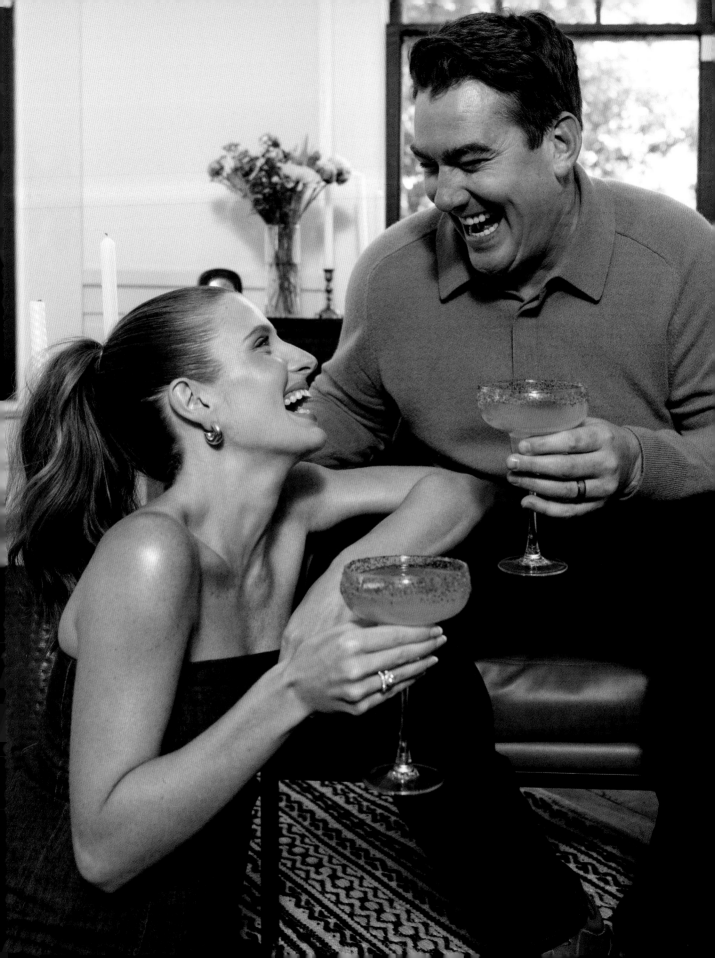

SPICY MARGARITA MOCKTAIL

Rachael: Before the world bombards you on what you can't and shouldn't have during pregnancy, let's focus on what you can have, and that's a delicious mocktail! Whether you drink alcohol or not, almost everyone can appreciate a refreshing and fun drink, and let's face it, there will be plenty of water to be had for the next 6 months. So slick your hair back, put on something you feel confident in, and put life on hold for a moment (because sometimes a moment is all we have).

SERVINGS: 2	PREP TIME: 5 MINUTES	TOTAL TIME: 7 MINUTES

Juice of 5 limes
Juice of 1 lemon
Juice of 1 navel orange
2 tablespoons agave syrup
½ teaspoon Tajin seasoning
Ice cubes
2 ounces zero-proof nonalcoholic
  tequila, optional

FOR THE GLASSES
Tajin seasoning to rim glass
1 small lime, cut in wedges
½ fresh jalapeño, sliced
Ice cubes

1 Add all the ingredients to a cocktail shaker and shake vigorously for 30 seconds.

2 **Prepare the margarita glasses.** Add Tajin in a shallow dish, enough to cover the bottom. Moisten the rims of the glasses with a lime wedge and dip the glass rims into the Tajin seasoning. Add sliced jalapeños to the margarita glass and top with more ice.

3 Strain the mixture into the prepared margarita glasses. Garnish with an additional sprinkle of Tajin and a lime wedge before serving.

Note   *Our favorite brand of nonalcoholic tequila is Ritual. If a traditional margarita is desired instead, add 2 ounces of tequila to the shaker.*

CILANTRO-LIME COCONUT CHICKEN

Rachael: This picture makes me salivate just looking at it. The way a creamy sauce over chicken and rice would make my pregnancy cravings go haywire is unmatched. The flavor combination of cilantro, lime, and coconut milk mixes Southeast Asian and Latin American influences, creating the perfect fusion dish. And let's face it, I know I can't be the only one out here with a rice addiction during pregnancy. Give me all the recipes over rice!

SERVINGS: 4	PREP TIME: 10 MINUTES	TOTAL TIME: 35 MINUTES

4 boneless, skinless chicken breasts
Salt and pepper, to taste
2 tablespoons coconut oil
½ teaspoon red pepper flakes
3 garlic cloves, minced
1 tablespoon grated fresh ginger
½ teaspoon ground cumin
¼ teaspoon ground turmeric
¼ cup chopped fresh cilantro
Zest and juice of 2 limes
1 cup full-fat canned coconut milk

SERVING OPTIONS
Cooked basmati rice
Cooked quinoa
Roasted vegetables
Fresh lime wedges
Chopped fresh cilantro
Sliced avocado
Cherry tomato halves

1 Season the chicken breasts with salt and pepper on both sides.

2 In a large skillet, heat the coconut oil over medium-high heat. Once hot, add the chicken breasts to the skillet and cook for 5 to 6 minutes on each side or until golden brown. Remove the chicken from the skillet and set aside on a plate.

3 In the same skillet, add the red pepper flakes, garlic, ginger, cumin, and turmeric with additional salt and pepper. Sauté for 1 to 2 minutes or until fragrant. Stir in the cilantro, lime zest, lime juice, and coconut milk. Bring the mixture to a simmer.

4 Return the cooked chicken breasts to the skillet, nestling them into the sauce. Reduce the heat to low and let the chicken simmer in the sauce for 5 to 7 minutes, allowing the flavors to meld together and the chicken to absorb some of the sauce.

5 Once the chicken is fully cooked with an internal temperature of 165°F (74°C), and the sauce has reduced slightly, remove the skillet from the heat.

6 Serve the chicken over rice, quinoa, or roasted vegetables. Drizzle some of the pan sauce over the chicken. Garnish the chicken with sliced lime wedges, chopped cilantro, avocado slices, or cherry tomatoes, if desired.

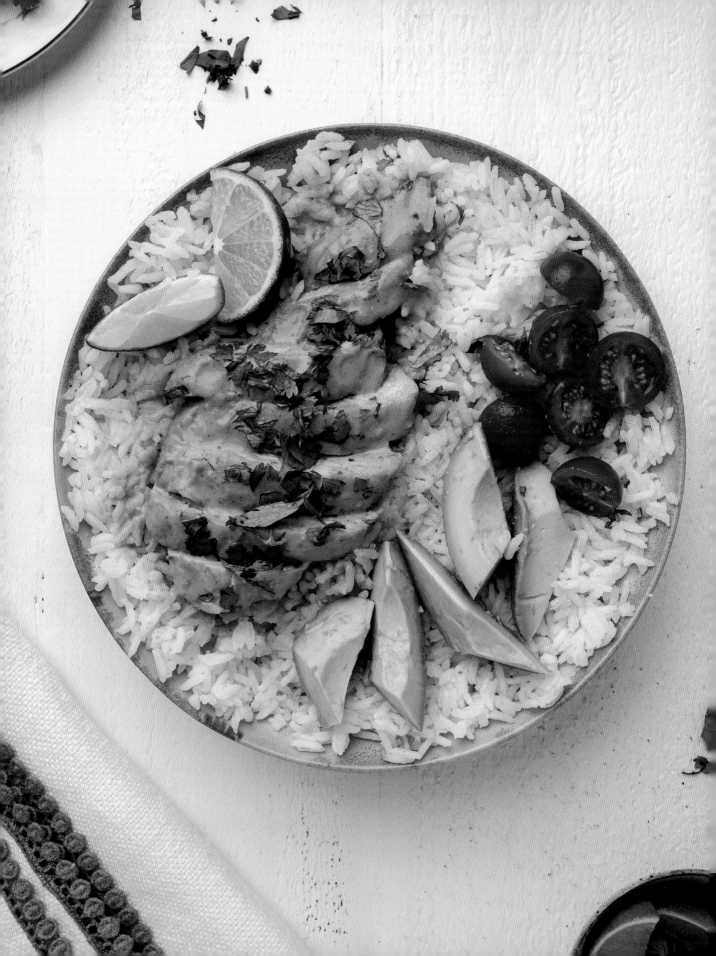

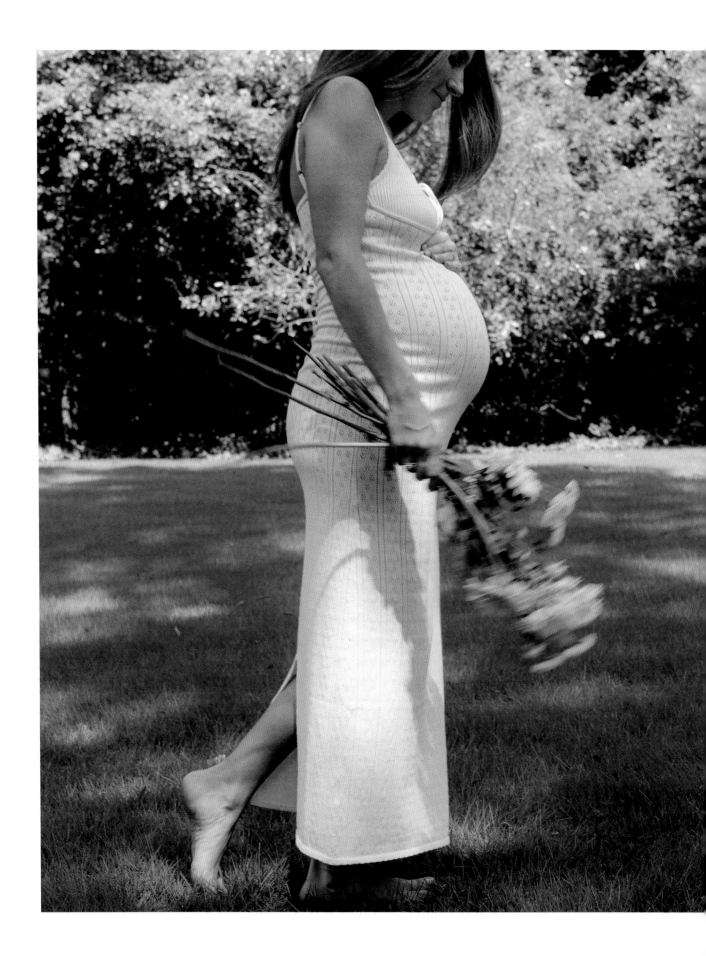

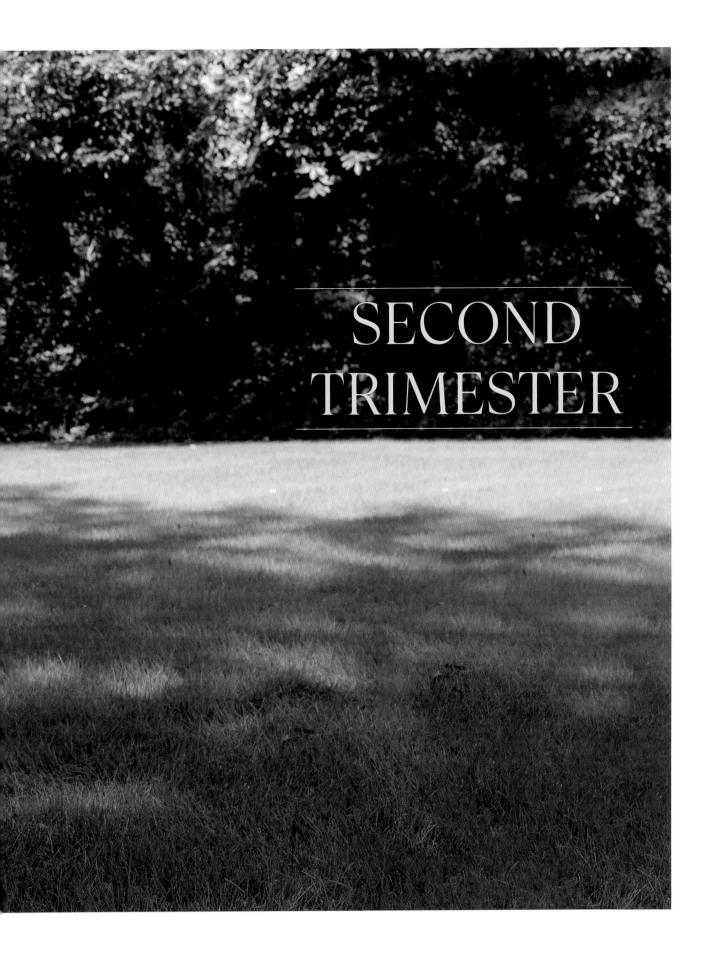

SECOND
TRIMESTER

*W*elcome to the second trimester. Although I can't promise all smooth sailing, during the next 15 weeks of your pregnancy you should start to feel some relief on all those lingering early pregnancy symptoms. They call it the "honeymoon period" for a good reason (not just because the sex is better). In the first trimester, there are a lot of unknowns, doctor visits, and things to be confirmed in regard to your baby's health and well-being. It can be a scary and overwhelming time. The second trimester brings another shift in your mental and emotional state, allowing your body and mind to take a deep breath from the fears and anxiety you had during the first trimester. Physically, your body is also shifting as your nausea and fatigue are lessening and your energy levels are starting to increase. You are still growing a human, so be kind to yourself, but our hope for you is that you can find some enjoyment in this stage of pregnancy.

SECOND TRIMESTER MILESTONES

- Your baby's eyes are starting to move by now (or will very soon) and they can begin to see light, so limit your screen time. Wink!

- Your little one may now be bouncing, flipping, and turning around to show off their new skill of being able to move their joints. It's an early sign of the lively personality that's already beginning to shine through, and they're saying, "I'm here and I'm growing, and here comes a kick to the ribs!"

- The unique fingerprint of your little baby is now starting to take shape. It's the tiny detail that will literally set them apart from everyone else in the world.

- The eyebrows, eyelashes, lips, and fingernails of your baby have formed by this point. It's almost like they are getting ready for their debut.

- Your baby may now be sucking their thumb in the uterus and sometimes you may catch it on an ultrasound! They're already practicing their own self-soothing skills. Let's hope they use them often in those first months!

SYMPTOMS YOU MAY EXPERIENCE

- Decreasing fatigue (Hooray!)
- Fetal movement (aka the best feeling ever)
- Bloating and gas (Pregnancy farts are on another level, so beware.)
- Leg cramps
- Continued breast growth and less breast tenderness
- Your innie belly button becoming an outie
- Backaches
- Increasing appetite (Finally!)
- Swelling of the feet and hands

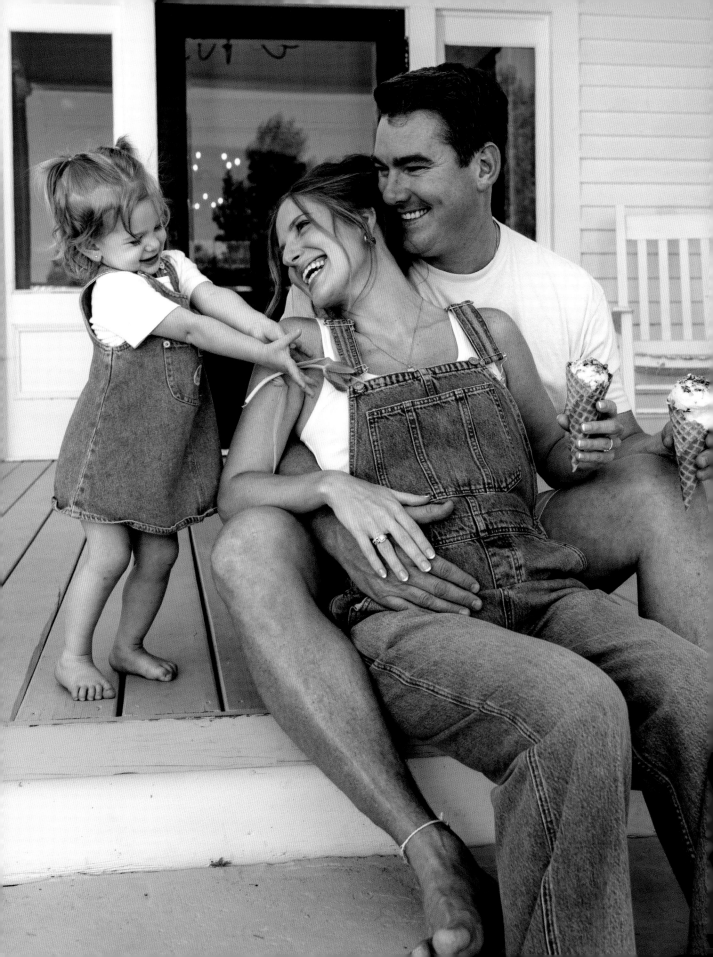

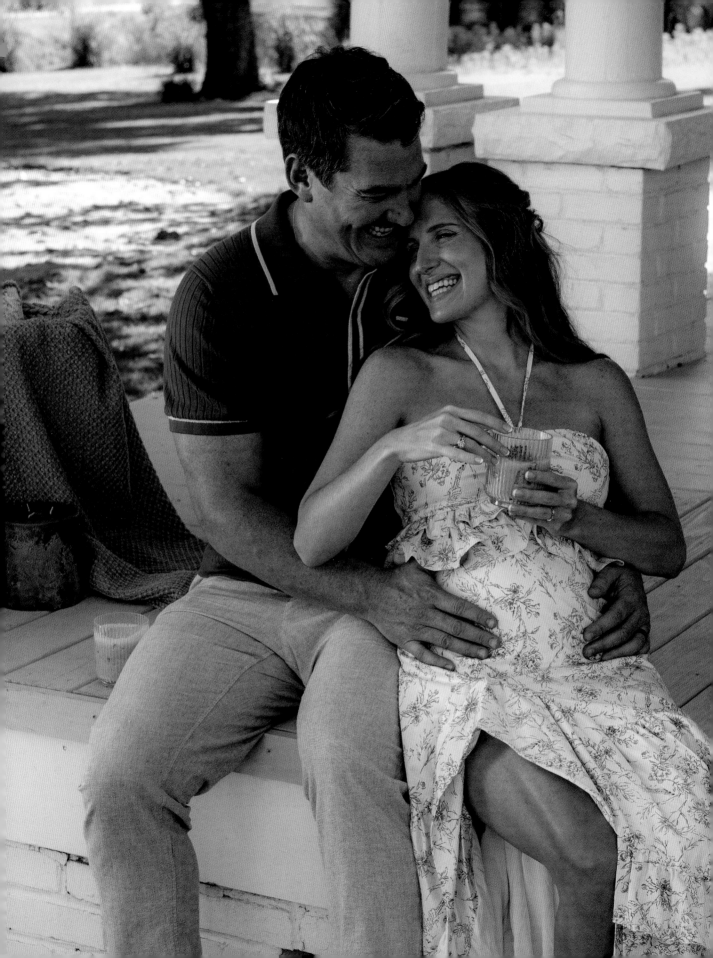

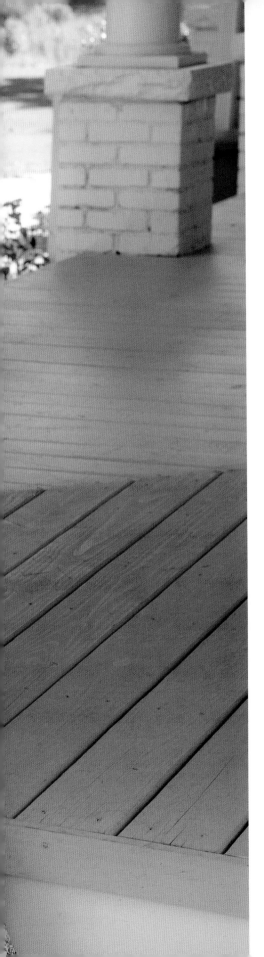

PREPARING FOR THIS SEASON

Transitioning into the second trimester means a season of growth, preparation, and deeper connection with both your baby and yourself. Yes, that finally means your bump will look less like a food baby and more like an actual baby. With that growth comes movement and those first few kicks that will lead to a deeper emotional connection between the two of you, becoming one of the most defining moments of your pregnancy. This may also be a season of bonding with your partner.

Some of my favorite things this season include planning a babymoon, however that looks for you. Whether it's a night away or a weekend out of town, celebrate each other or just yourself and this new adventure of parenthood you are about to embark on. Spoil yourself! Whether that's with passes to your favorite workout classes or a prenatal massage, do something for you. If you are finding out the gender of your sweet baby, now is the perfect time to plan a gender-reveal party with your loved ones and prepare your registry for all the things you have no idea you need but you will soon find out why you do!

GRILLED PEACH-BASIL GOAT CHEESE SANDWICHES

Rachael: A sweet, creamy, savory bite is what you're going to experience when you try this grilled cheese. A simple recipe that transports you to the sweetness of summer. It's giving *Hamptons in June with a private chef who is preparing a simple lunch before dinner* vibes. As I type this, 29-weeks pregnant in the month of June, I would give anything to be there, but for now, this sandwich will do.

SERVINGS: 2	PREP TIME: 5 MINUTES	TOTAL TIME: 12 MINUTES

4 ounces (113g) goat cheese, softened
4 slices gluten-free bread of choice
Handful of fresh basil leaves
1 ripe fresh peach, halved and thinly sliced
Pinch of salt and pepper
2 tablespoons honey
2 tablespoons olive oil or butter

1 Heat a skillet over medium-low heat.

2 Spread the softened goat cheese evenly onto two slices of bread.

3 Arrange the basil leaves and then the peach slices on top of the goat cheese, and season with a pinch of salt and pepper.

4 Drizzle 1 tablespoon of honey over the peach and basil layers on each slice of bread.

5 Close the two sandwiches with the remaining slices of bread.

6 Add olive oil to the warm skillet and swirl the skillet to coat the entire cooking surface.

7 Carefully place the assembled sandwiches in the skillet. Cook the sandwiches for 3 to 4 minutes on each side or until the bread is golden brown and crispy and the goat cheese is melted.

8 Remove the grilled sandwiches from the skillet and let them cool for 2 minutes before slicing diagonally and serving immediately.

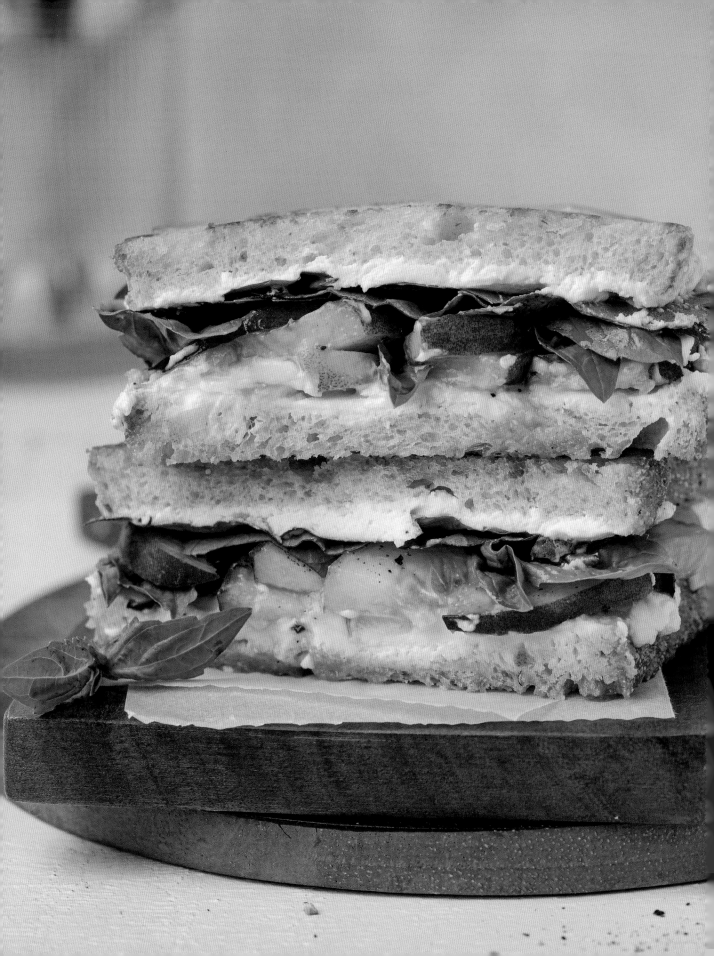

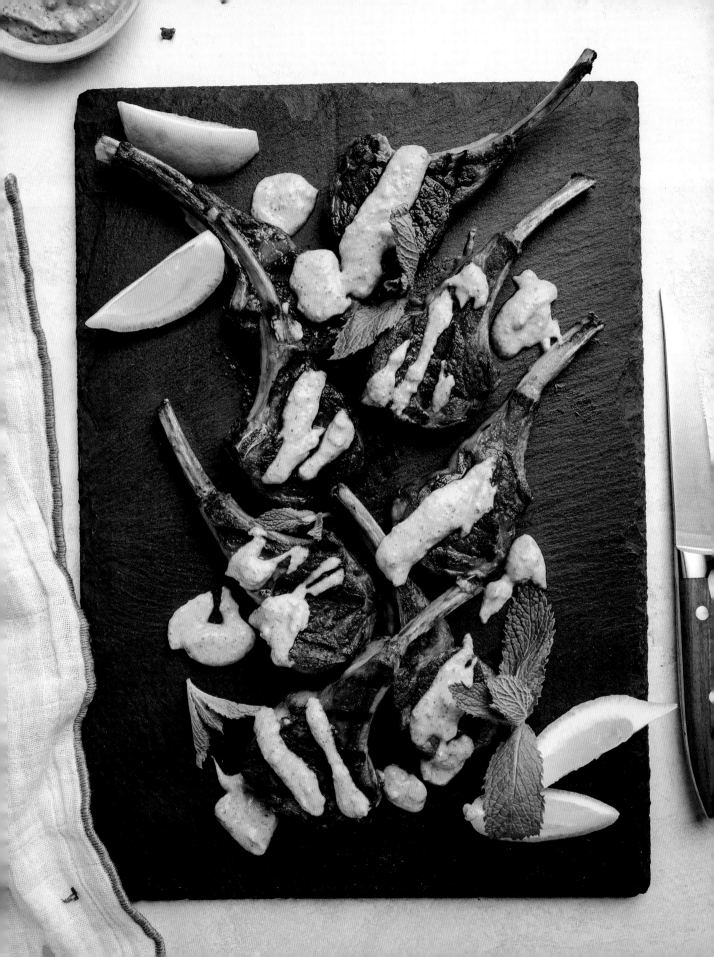

LAMB

WITH PEACH & MINT PESTO

Rachael: Pregnancy aside, if there is one dish you want to add to your recipe roster that will be sure to impress dinner guests, it's these lollipop lamb chops! Tom started making lollipop lamb years ago, and I thought that it was just something you ordered at a 5-star restaurant. Turns out they are super simple to prepare, It just takes confidence to execute. Pair them with the peach-and-mint pesto and you can basically call yourself a Michelin chef.

SERVINGS: 4	PREP TIME: 20 MINUTES	TOTAL TIME: 30 MINUTES

6-8 lollipop (frenched) or regular lamb chops, ¾-1 inch (2-2.5cm) thick
Salt and pepper, to taste
3 tablespoons olive oil, divided
2 ripe fresh peaches, peeled, halved, and pitted
¼ cup fresh mint leaves, plus more for garnish, optional
2 garlic cloves
¼ cup almonds or pine nuts, toasted
Zest and juice of 1 lemon

1 Let the lamb chops come to room temperature. Season lamb with salt and pepper on both sides and brush them with 1 tablespoon of olive oil.

2 Preheat the grill to medium-high heat. If you don't have a grill, the lamb can be seared in a pan over medium-high heat with a little more olive oil.

3 Cook the lamb on the grill for about 3 to 4 minutes per side or until 130°F (55°C) for medium-rare or to your desired level of doneness. Make sure to watch for flare-ups so your chops don't burn—lamb is prone to this.

4 Once cooked to your desired doneness, transfer the lamb from the grill to a baking sheet with a wire rack to rest for about 10 minutes.

5 To peel the peaches, use a vegetable peeler, or score the skin and drop them into boiling water for 30 to 40 seconds, then remove and rinse in cold water; the skin comes off easily.

6 In a food processor or blender, combine the peaches, mint leaves, garlic cloves, almonds, lemon zest, lemon juice, and the remaining 2 tablespoons of olive oil, and blend until smooth and well combined. Add additional salt and pepper to taste. If the pesto is too thick, you can add a little more olive oil to thin it out.

7 Transfer the grilled or pan-seared lamb to serving plates. Spoon the peach-and-mint pesto over the lamb, dividing it evenly among the servings.

8 Garnish the lamb with additional fresh mint leaves, if desired, and serve.

PEACH-COBBLER COOKIES

Rachael: We were originally going to do a classic peach cobbler recipe for the book. On the night that we sat down as a team to review the recipes, my pregnant self was craving cookies, and we realized we didn't have a cookie recipe in the book. Thus, the peach-cobbler cookies were born. It's a treat that will last the entire week unless you have no self-control, like me, and plan on eating all of them in one sitting.

SERVINGS: 12	PREP TIME: 15 MINUTES	TOTAL TIME: 30 MINUTES

2 cups almond flour

¼ cup coconut flour

¼ cup plus a pinch coconut sugar or granulated sweetener of your choice

1 teaspoon baking powder

¼ teaspoon salt

¼ cup coconut oil, melted

¼ cup almond milk or milk of choice

1 large egg

1 tablespoon honey

1 teaspoon vanilla extract

1 cup diced fresh peaches, about 2 medium peaches

½ teaspoon ground cinnamon

1 Preheat the oven to 350°F (180°C) and line a baking sheet with parchment paper.

2 In a large bowl, whisk together the almond flour, coconut flour, ¼ cup coconut sugar, baking powder, and salt until well combined.

3 In a small bowl, whisk together the melted coconut oil, almond milk, egg, honey and vanilla extract until smooth.

4 Pour the wet ingredients into the bowl with the dry ingredients and mix until a dough forms. If the dough seems too dry, you can add a little more almond milk, one tablespoon at a time, until the dough comes together. If the dough is too wet, add more almond flour.

5 Gently fold in the diced peaches until evenly distributed throughout the dough.

6 Using a cookie scoop or spoon, drop rounded tablespoons of dough onto the prepared baking sheet, spacing them about 2 inches apart. Use your hands to gently flatten each cookie slightly.

7 In a small bowl, mix the ground cinnamon and a pinch of coconut sugar. Sprinkle this mixture over the tops of the cookies.

8 Bake the cookies in the preheated oven for 12 to 15 minutes or until the edges are golden brown.

9 Allow the cookies to cool on the baking sheet for a few minutes before transferring them to a wire rack to cool completely.

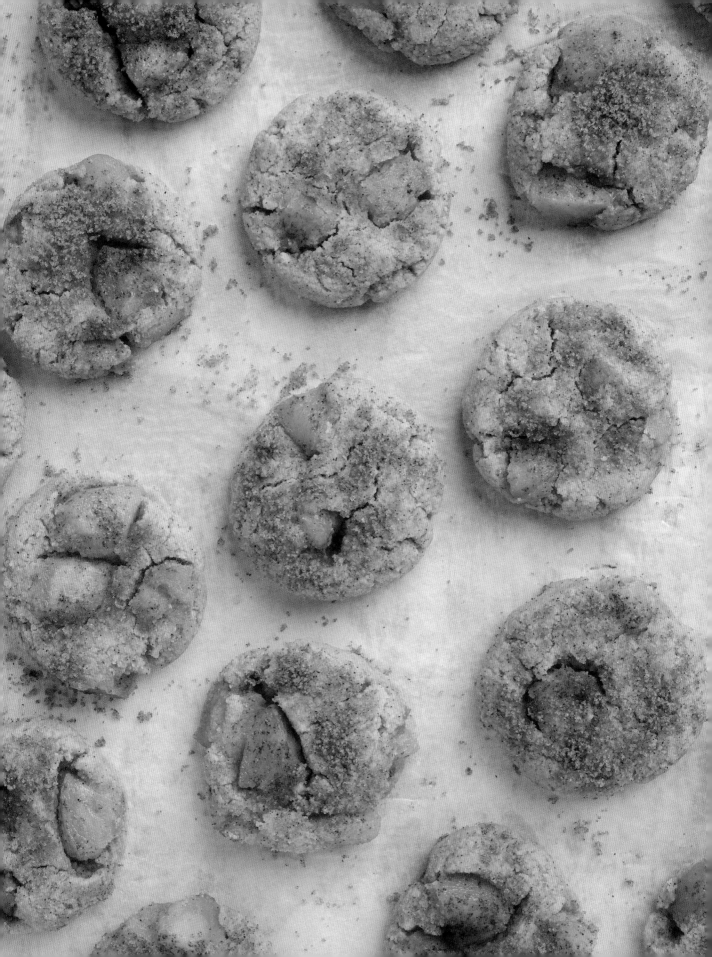

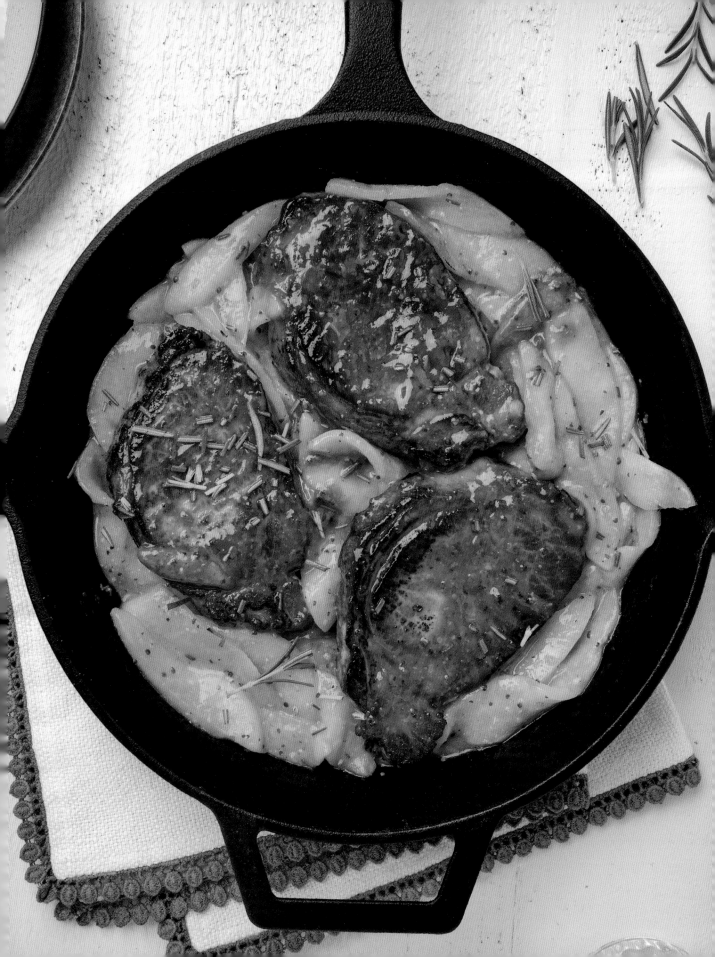

PEAR-MOSTARDA PORK CHOPS

Rachael: We are getting creative with how to utilize pears for this recipe, giving you a dish you've probably never tried—or even heard of, for that matter. A *mostarda* is an Italian condiment that's made with fruit and mustard oil. We used pear and a mixture of Dijon and whole-grain mustards to bring our own version of mostarda to life. Now, pregnancy does strange things to your taste buds, so half of you may think this sounds amazing and the other half may be completely turned off by the description of it, to which I say, to each their own.

SERVINGS: 2–4	**PREP TIME:** 10 MINUTES	**TOTAL TIME:** 30 MINUTES

4 boneless pork chops ½-¾ inch (1.25-2cm) thick
Salt and pepper, to taste
2 tablespoons olive oil
2 fresh pears, peeled, cored, and sliced ⅛-inch thick
¼ cup apple cider vinegar
2 tablespoons honey
1 tablespoon Dijon mustard
1 tablespoon whole-grain mustard
1 teaspoon finely chopped fresh rosemary, plus more to garnish, optional
¼ cup chicken or vegetable broth

1 Let the pork chops come to room temperature and season them generously with salt and pepper on both sides.

2 In a large skillet, heat the olive oil over medium-high heat.

3 Add the seasoned pork chops to the skillet and sear them for 3 to 4 minutes on each side or until golden brown and the internal temperature reaches 140°F (60°C). Remove the pork chops from the skillet and set them aside on a plate.

4 In the same skillet, add the sliced pears and cook for 2 to 3 minutes or until they begin to soften.

5 Add the apple cider vinegar, honey, Dijon mustard, whole-grain mustard, and chopped rosemary to the skillet with the pears. Stir to combine.

6 Allow the sauce to simmer for 2 to 3 minutes or until it begins to reduce slightly.

7 Pour in the chicken broth and stir to combine the sauce.

8 Return the seared pork chops to the skillet, nestling them into the sauce.

9 Reduce the heat to low and let the pork chops simmer in the sauce for another 5 to 7 minutes or until they are heated through and the sauce has reduced.

10 Transfer the pork chops to serving plates. Spoon the sauce and pears over the pork chops and garnish with additional finely chopped rosemary, if desired.

PEAR & PROSCIUTTO POPPERS

Rachael: I feel pretty lucky to have a husband who makes whatever random pregnancy cravings I have a reality, and I feel even luckier to be able to share that with all of you. These pear and prosciutto poppers stemmed from my prosciutto-wrapped melon obsession while we were in Italy. Salty meat with a ripe fruit just does something to me. In Tom fashion, we added a mixture to drizzle over the top because he believes life is just better with sauces.

SERVINGS: 2–4	**PREP TIME**: 35 MINUTES	**TOTAL TIME**: 1 HOUR

2 firm, ripe fresh pears, cut into bite-size wedges or cubes

½ pound (227g) prosciutto slices, cut in half

Toothpicks, soaked in water for 30 minutes

FOR THE SAUCE

2 tablespoons honey

¼ teaspoon vanilla extract

Pinch of ground cinnamon

Pinch of salt

FOR SERVING

Arugula or mixed greens

¼ cup chopped walnuts or pecans

4 ounces (113g) goat cheese, crumbled

Balsamic or fig glaze, optional

1 Wash the pears thoroughly and pat them dry with a paper towel. Cut the pears into bite-size wedges or cubes, discarding the stems, seeds, and cores.

2 Preheat the oven to 375°F (190°C). Wrap each pear wedge with half a piece of prosciutto. Secure the prosciutto to the pears using the water-soaked toothpicks. Place the wrapped pears on a baking sheet lined with parchment paper and bake for 22 to 25 minutes.

3 **Prepare the suace.** Mix the honey, vanilla, cinnamon and salt together in a small bowl.

4 **To serve,** on a serving platter, create a bed of arugula. Remove the prosciutto-wrapped pears from the oven, and arrange the pear poppers on the arugula. Drizzle the honey sauce over the poppers. Top with the walnuts and goat cheese. Drizzle with balsamic glaze, if desired.

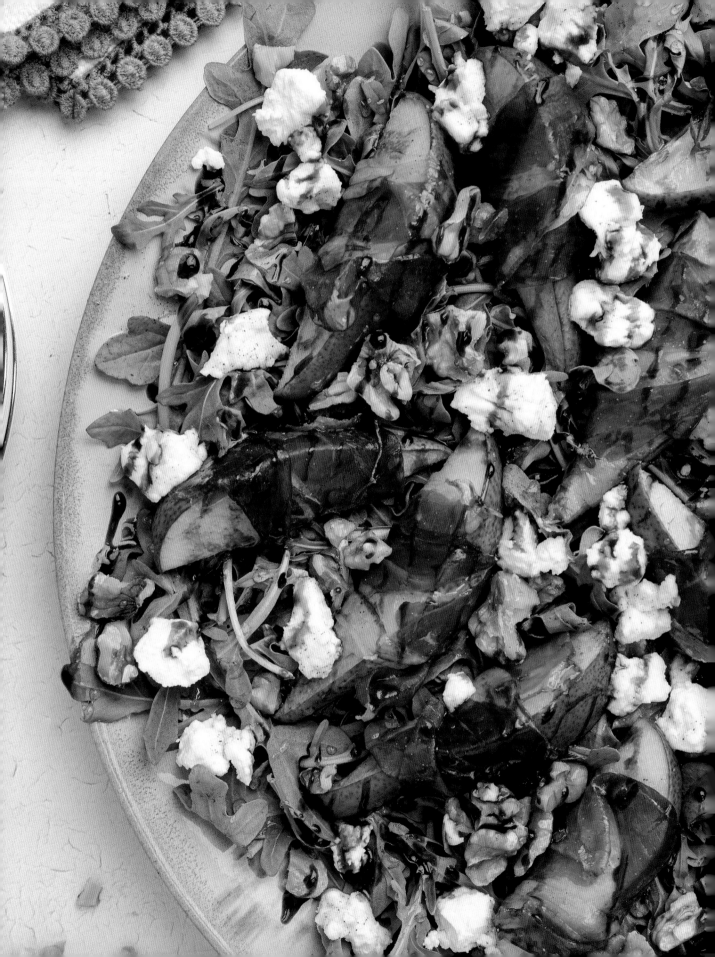

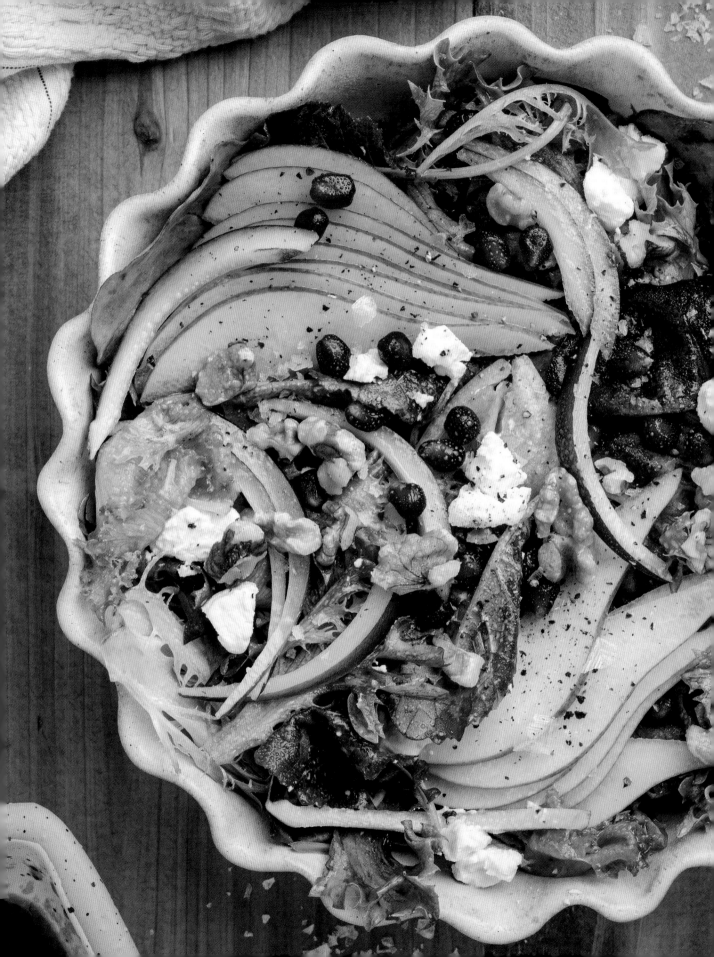

FALL-WINTER PEAR SALAD

Rachael: During my first pregnancy, I craved healthy food. The idea of salad and a smoothie made my mouth water, whereas in my second pregnancy, I craved anything I could sink my teeth into, like a fat, juicy burger. This recipe is a hybrid of those two cravings. It's a healthy salad that will help your body get the nutrients it needs, while also having a well-rounded bite to it. Whether you're delivering in winter, summer, spring, or fall, this salad does the trick.

SERVINGS: 2–4	PREP TIME: 10 MINUTES	TOTAL TIME: 10 MINUTES

4 cups mixed salad greens, such as arugula, spinach, and romaine

½ cup roughly chopped walnuts

¼ cup crumbled goat cheese, optional

¼ cup fresh pomegranate arils or dried cranberries

¼ cup thinly sliced red onion

¼ cup balsamic vinaigrette dressing or more to taste

Salt and pepper, to taste

2 ripe fresh pears

FOR BALSAMIC VINAIGRETTE

¼ cup balsamic vinegar

¾ cup olive oil

2 tablespoons honey

1 tablespoon Dijon mustard

½ teaspoon salt

½ teaspoon black pepper

1 garlic clove, finely minced or grated

1 **Prepare the balsamic vinaigrette.** Whisk all the vinaigrette ingredients together in a small bowl until combined. (See note.)

2 Thoroughly wash and dry the mixed salad greens. Place them in a large salad bowl.

3 Sprinkle the walnuts, goat cheese crumbles (if using), pomegranate arils, and sliced red onion over the salad. Drizzle ¼ cup of the dressing over the top, season with salt and pepper, and gently toss.

4 Core the pears and thinly slice them. Arrange the pear slices over the dressed salad greens.

5 Drizzle additional balsamic vinaigrette over the salad ingredients to taste.

Note   *This balsamic vinaigrette recipe yields about 1 cup of dressing. Store the extra dressing in an airtight container in the fridge for up to 2 weeks.*

APPLE NACHOS

Rachael: Apple nachos will be the healthiest nachos you've ever had. It's a recipe you'll come back to over and over again, especially when the little bun in your oven is old enough to want to help cook in the kitchen. Right now, our daughter is at the age where she wants her hands in everything and re-creating this recipe with her is not only playful and delicious, but it reminds us of the time we first prepared these when she was the size of an apple and we daydreamed about the moment when she would be old enough to help.

SERVINGS: 4–6	PREP TIME: 10 MINUTES	TOTAL TIME: 12 MINUTES

2 apples (we use Granny Smith or Honeycrisp)
1 cup vanilla Greek yogurt or vanilla cashew yogurt
Dash of ground cinnamon
¾ cup creamy almond butter
¼ cup granola
¼ cup chopped walnuts
¼ cup pomegranate arils
1 tablespoon toasted coconut flakes

1 Core the apples. We find an 8-slice standard apple corer is a bit thick, so we halve those to 16 slices.

2 Place the yogurt in the middle of a large serving plate, sprinkle a dash of cinnamon over the yogurt, and lay the apples over the yogurt, circling the plate and layering as you go. Drizzle almond butter over the apples to help the toppings stick. Then top with granola, walnuts, pomegranate arils, and coconut flakes. Dip and enjoy!

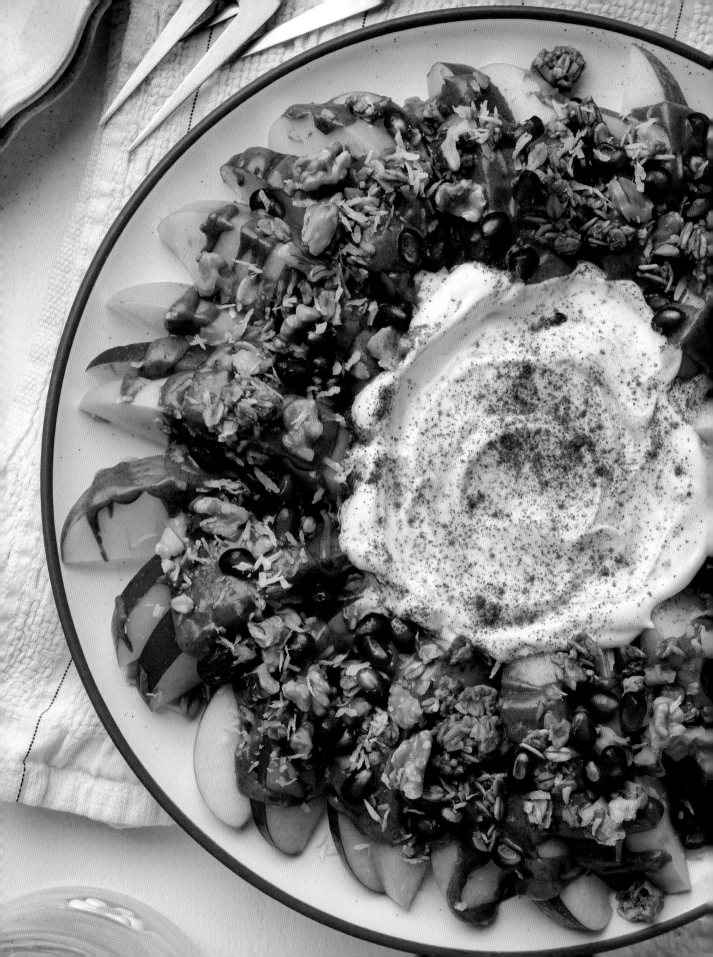

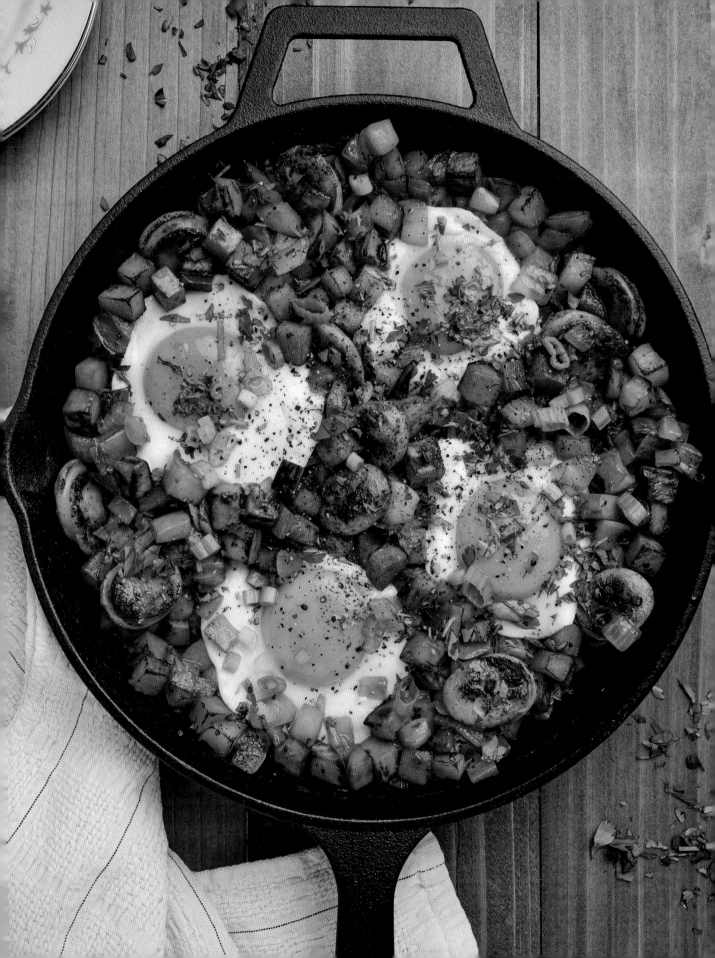

APPLE, SWEET POTATO & SAUSAGE BREAKFAST SKILLET

Rachael: Our breakfast skillet is a fan-favorite recipe from our first book, *Meals She Eats,* and to be honest, it's a fan favorite in the Sullivan household, too—we cook this whenever entertaining house guests for the weekend. We knew we had to incorporate a rendition of this recipe in this book, so we added a sweet take to a savory dish, incorporating the apples. Since I've been known to finish an entire skillet, portion control is unheard of when it comes to this recipe. After all, I'm eating for two, right?

SERVINGS: 4	PREP TIME: 10 MINUTES	TOTAL TIME: 45 MINUTES

1 tablespoon olive oil

1 pound (450g) chicken breakfast sausage patties or links (if links, cut into ¼-inch rounds)

1 large sweet potato, peeled and diced

1 large apple, cored and diced

1 small white onion, diced

2 garlic cloves, minced

1 teaspoon fresh thyme

1 tablespoon maple syrup

Salt and pepper, to taste

4 large eggs

SERVING OPTIONS

Chopped fresh parsley

Chopped green onions

Sprinkle of ground cinnamon

1 Heat olive oil in a large skillet over medium heat. Add the sausage and cook until browned and cooked through, about 8 to 10 minutes. Remove the cooked sausage from the skillet and set aside.

2 In the same skillet, add the diced sweet potato and additional olive oil if needed. Cook for 5 to 7 minutes, stirring occasionally, until the sweet potato begins to soften.

3 Add the apple, onion, garlic, thyme, and maple syrup to the skillet. Season with salt and pepper to taste. Cook for another 5 minutes or until the sweet potatoes and apples are tender.

4 Return the cooked sausage to the skillet and stir to combine with the sweet potatoes, apples, and onion. Cook for an additional 2 to 3 minutes to heat everything through.

5 Use a spoon to make four wells or indentations in the skillet mixture large enough to fit an egg, about 3 inches (7.5cm) each. Crack one egg into each well.

6 Cover the skillet and cook for 5 to 7 minutes or until the egg whites are set. If you prefer firmer yolks, cook them longer until desired doneness is reached.

7 Once the eggs are cooked, if you would like, garnish the breakfast skillet with chopped fresh parsley, green onions, and cinnamon before serving immediately from the skillet.

GREEN APPLE BLT

Rachael: I'm here to tell you that sandwiches are still a part of the pregnancy diet. I lived off of BLTs for both my pregnancies. Some days, admittedly, it was just bacon and bread but sometimes the baby wants what the baby wants. Apples are a fun way to add a bit of crisp texture and sweetness to the sandwich, and you know what they say, "an apple a day keeps the doctor away" or in our case, positive news during our monthly baby checkups.

SERVINGS: 2	PREP TIME: 10 MINUTES	TOTAL TIME: 18 MINUTES

4-6 slices bacon
4 bread slices, your choice (we prefer gluten-free)
1 ripe avocado, sliced
Salt and pepper, to taste
1 green apple, cored and thinly sliced
½ heirloom tomato, thinly sliced
1 cup arugula
1 tablespoon mayonnaise
1 tablespoon honey-mustard sauce

1 In a medium skillet over medium high heat, cook your bacon slices for 7-8 minutes flipping once or twice. Remove from heat.

2 While the bacon cooks, toast the bread slices in a toaster until golden brown and crispy.

3 In a small bowl, mash the ripe avocado slices with a fork until smooth. Season with salt and pepper to taste. Spread a layer of mashed avocado on two of the toasted bread slices.

4 Layer each sandwich evenly with half of the green apple slices, 2 to 3 bacon slices, tomato slices, and ½ cup of arugula. Season with salt and pepper to taste..

5 In second small bowl, mix together the mayonnaise and honey mustard. Spread 1 tablespoon of the mayo-mustard mixture onto each of the remaining two bread slices and then place on top of the arugula.

6 Use a sharp knife to slice each sandwich in half diagonally before serving.

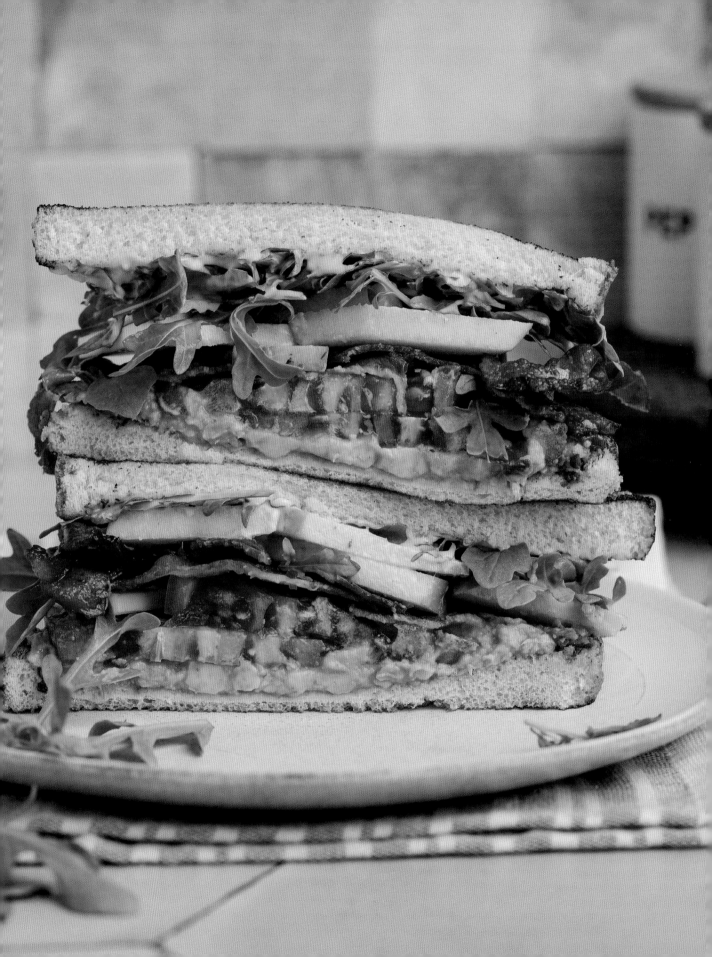

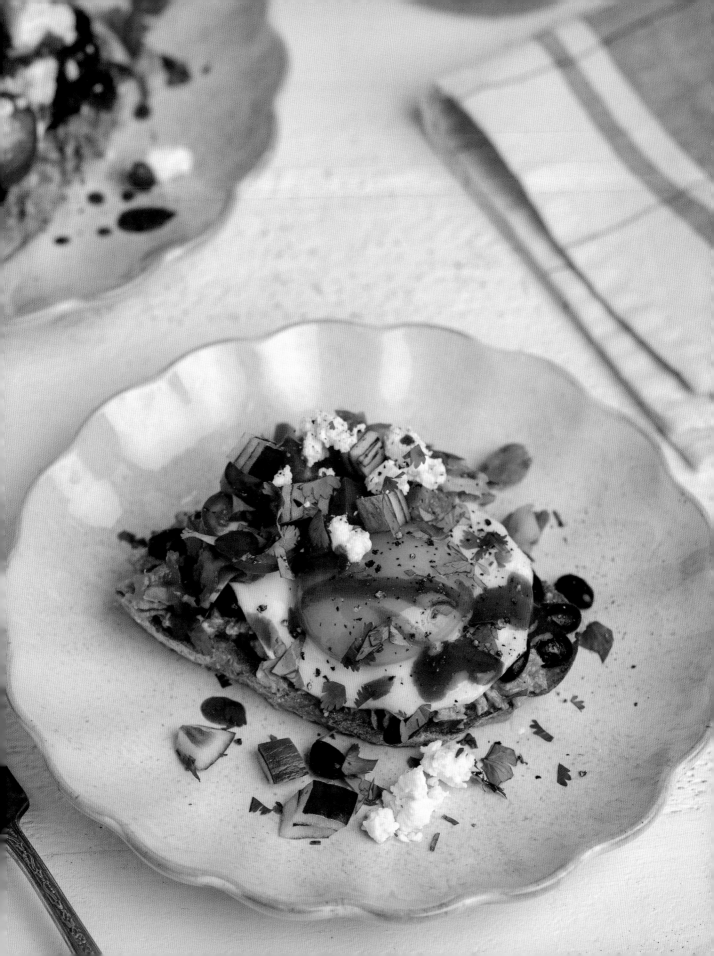

AVOCADO HUEVOS RANCHEROS TOAST

Rachael: We love Mexican-inspired dishes. Our babymoon was in Cabo San Lucas, half because of the beach, but mainly because the room service had authentic tacos I could order whenever my little pregnant self desired ... which was at all hours of the day. For breakfast, I loved eating a rendition of this huevos rancheros toast because it took avocado toast to the next level. Please enjoy all of my favorite flavors packed into one dish.

SERVINGS: 2	PREP TIME: 10 MINUTES	TOTAL TIME: 15 MINUTES

1 ripe avocado
½ teaspoon chili powder
½ teaspoon garlic powder
½ teaspoon ground cumin
Juice of ½ lime
Salt and pepper, to taste
2 slices gluten-free bread of choice
1 tablespoon olive oil
2 large eggs
½ cup black beans, drained and rinsed
¼ cup salsa
¼ cup diced red onion
¼ cup chopped fresh cilantro

SERVING OPTIONS
Hot sauce
Cotija cheese

1 Cut the avocado in half, remove the pit, and scoop the flesh into a small bowl. Mash the avocado with a fork until smooth. Thoroughly mix the avocado together with the chili powder, garlic powder, cumin, and lime juice and then season with salt and pepper to taste.

2 Toast the gluten-free bread slices until golden brown and crispy.

3 Heat the olive oil in a medium nonstick skillet over medium heat. Crack the eggs into the skillet and cook 3 to 4 minutes until the whites are set but the yolks are still runny or cook to your desired level of doneness. Season with salt and pepper.

4 Spread a generous amount of mashed avocado onto each toasted bread slice.

5 On each toast slice, spoon ¼ cup of the black beans over the mashed avocado and then follow with 1/8 cup of the salsa.

6 Carefully place a cooked egg on top of each toast slice.

7 Garnish each slice equally with diced red onion and chopped cilantro.

8 If desired, top with hot sauce and cotija cheese.

9 Serve immediately while the eggs are still warm.

— week 16 —

MINT CHOCOLATE CHIP AVOCADO ICE CREAM

Rachael: We made this recipe when our daughter Sutton was the size of an avocado. It always stuck out to me as such a fun week to celebrate because there is an underlying joy that comes with an evening scoop of ice cream, especially if it has chocolate chips in it. I knew when we first started outlining the book that I couldn't wait to do a lifestyle shoot that incorporated Sutton with this ice cream recipe, because it holds such a special place in my heart. I love that we'll always have these photos to look back on now.

SERVINGS: 4–6	**PREP TIME:** 7 MINUTES	**TOTAL TIME:** 5 HOURS 20 MINUTES OR OVERNIGHT TO FREEZE

2 large avocados, halved, pitted, and peeled.
1 frozen ripe banana (peel and place in freezer at least 1 hour)
Juice of 1 lemon
3 tablespoons maple syrup or honey
1 (14-ounce/397g) can full-fat coconut milk
5–7 fresh mint leaves
Pinch of salt
1 cup dark chocolate morsels

SERVING OPTIONS
Gluten-free sugar cones
Toasted coconut flakes
Crushed pistachios

1 Place a medium metal bowl or loaf pan in the freezer to chill.

2 Place avocado, banana, lemon juice, maple syrup, coconut milk, mint leaves, and a pinch of salt into a blender and blend until well incorporated and creamy.

3 Remove the bowl from the freezer and pour the mixture into the bowl. Fold in the chocolate chips.

4 Cover the bowl with plastic wrap and return to the freezer. Freeze for at least 4 hours or overnight. When ready to serve, remove from the freezer and let sit at room temperature for 10 minutes to soften. Either serve ice cream in a bowl or cone and top with coconut flakes and crushed pistachios, if desired.

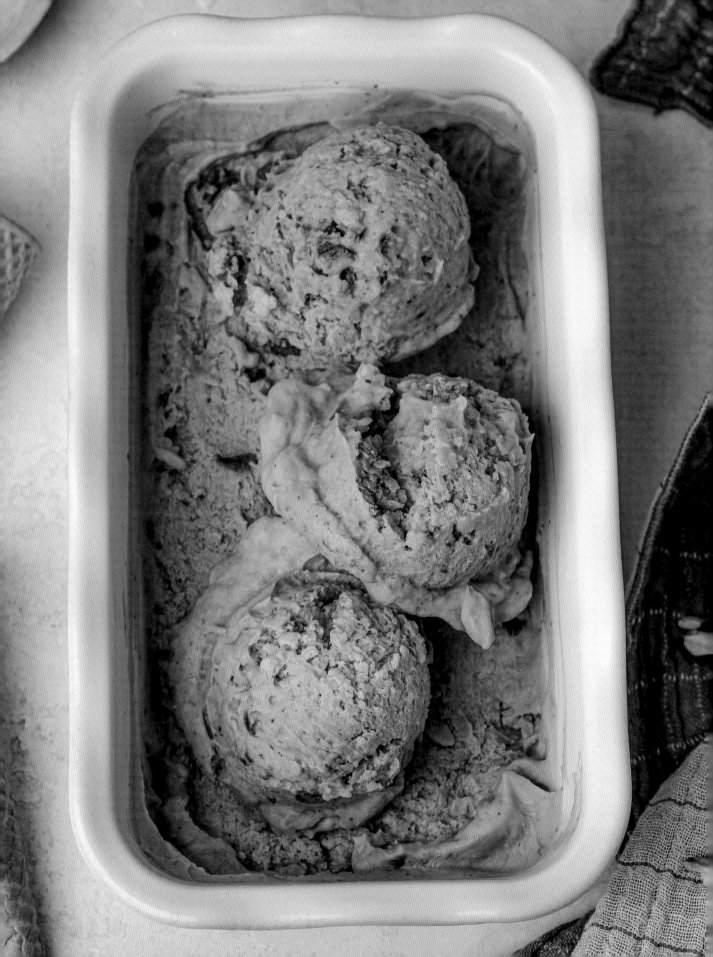

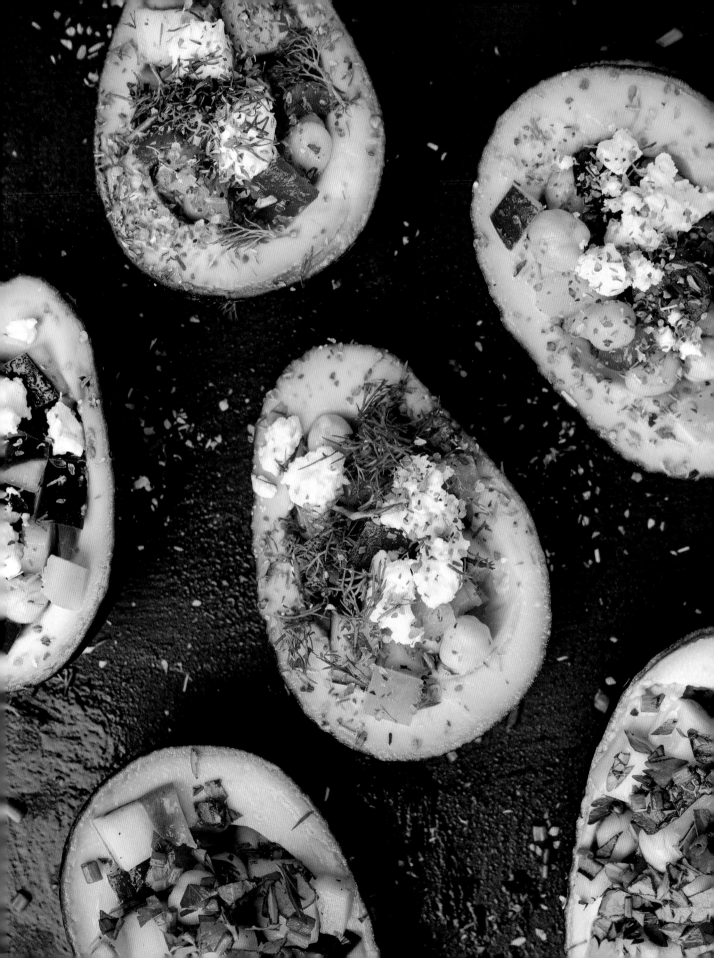

MEDITERRANEAN CHICKPEA AVOCADO BOATS, THREE WAYS

Rachael: There is a shift happening at this point during pregnancy. Your sex drive may start to heighten after a long first trimester hiatus, which may or may not be the reason for that pregnancy glow. Either way, things are looking and feeling brighter, so we want to make sure we nourish you with foods that give off that same energy! These stuffed avocado boats are filled with ingredients that are good for you and will enhance that glow, instead of making you feel like grease is oozing out of your pores.

SERVINGS: 2–4	PREP TIME: 20 MINUTES	TOTAL TIME: 20 MINUTES

2 ripe avocados
1 (14-ounce/397g) can chickpeas, drained and rinsed
¼ cup diced cucumber
¼ cup diced tomato
¼ cup diced red onion
¼ cup diced bell pepper, red or yellow
2 tablespoons chopped fresh parsley
2 tablespoons chopped fresh mint
2 tablespoons crumbled feta cheese, optional
Juice of 1 lemon
2 tablespoons extra-virgin olive oil
Salt and pepper, to taste

CLASSIC KALAMATA OLIVE TOPPINGS
¼ cup chopped Kalamata olives, pits removed
¼ cup crumbled feta cheese
¼ teaspoon dried oregano

GREEK-INSPIRED TOPPINGS
¼ cup diced tomato
2 tablespoons chopped fresh dill
2 tablespoons crumbled feta cheese
¼ teaspoon dried oregano

LEMON-HERB GREMOLATA TOPPINGS
Zest of 1 lemon
2 tablespoons chopped fresh basil
2 tablespoons chopped fresh cilantro
2 tablespoons chopped fresh chives
1 tablespoon olive oil

1 Halve the avocados lengthwise and remove the pits. Scoop out a little extra flesh from each avocado half to create a larger cavity for the filling. Dice the avocado that was scooped out and add it to a large mixing bowl.

2 In a large mixing bowl with the diced avocado, combine the chickpeas, cucumber, tomatoes, red onion, bell pepper, parsley, mint, and feta cheese (if using). Add lemon juice, extra-virgin olive oil, and salt and pepper to taste, and toss well to combine.

3 Divide the chickpea salad mixture evenly among the hollowed-out avocado halves, mounding it generously on top.

4 Customize the avocado boats to your liking by adding the toppings for any of the three variations.

ENDIVE CUPS, THREE WAYS

Tom: Have you ever heard of an endive? I had not when I was looking for a unique appetizer I could bring to a pool party. I wanted something that was fun, refreshing, and delicious. Pinterest then introduced me to this nutritious, crisp, and versatile vegetable. I will admit I was worried, since I had never heard of it, that I would have to find some specialty grocery store. Lucky for all of us, this is not the case, and every grocery store I have checked for it has been a successful trip. So, enjoy these endive cups (poolside, if possible)!

SERVINGS: 4–6	**PREP TIME:** 10 MINUTES	**TOTAL TIME:** 15 OR 40 MINUTES

2–3 Belgian endive heads

AVOCADO SALAD CUPS
2 ripe avocados, diced
1 small red onion, finely diced
1 heirloom tomato, diced
Juice of 1 lime
Salt and pepper, to taste

CHICKEN & DATE SALAD CUPS
1 pound (450g) boneless, skinless chicken breasts, cooked and shredded
½ cup chopped pitted dates
¼ cup olive oil
2 tablespoons chopped fresh parsley
2 tablespoons chopped fresh mint
Juice of 1 lemon
Salt and pepper, to taste

ROASTED ROOT VEGETABLE CUPS
2 medium carrots, peeled and diced
2 parsnips, peeled and diced
1 sweet potato, peeled and diced
2 tablespoons olive oil
Salt and pepper, to taste
¼ cup pomegranate juice
1 tablespoon balsamic vinegar
1 teaspoon honey or maple syrup
¼ cup pomegranate arils

Slice the root-end off each endive head and peel the larger leaves off to use for the cups. Try to find leaves about 4 to 6 inches long. Set aside and continue with your chosen recipe.

FOR AVOCADO SALAD CUPS
1 In a small bowl, combine the avocado, onion, tomato, and lime juice. Season with salt and pepper to taste. Gently toss to combine.
2 Spoon the avocado salad mixture into the endive cups. Serve and enjoy.

FOR CHICKEN & DATE SALAD CUPS
1 In a small bowl, combine the chicken, dates, olive oil, parsley, mint, and lemon juice. Season with salt and pepper to taste. Mix well to combine.
2 Spoon the chicken and date mixture into the endive cups. Serve and enjoy.

FOR ROASTED ROOT VEGETABLE CUPS
1 Preheat the oven to 400°F (200°C).
2 Line a large baking sheet with parchment paper. On the baking sheet, toss the carrots, parsnips, and sweet potato with olive oil, salt, and pepper until evenly coated and spread in a single layer.
3 Roast for 20 to 25 minutes or until the vegetables are tender and lightly caramelized.
4 Meanwhile, in a small saucepan, combine the pomegranate juice, vinegar, and honey. Simmer over medium heat, stirring occasionally, for 5 to 7 minutes, until the sauce has reduced and coats the back of a spoon.
5 Fill the endive cups with the roasted root vegetables and drizzle the pomegranate sauce over the top. Garnish with pomegranate arils, if desired. Serve and enjoy.

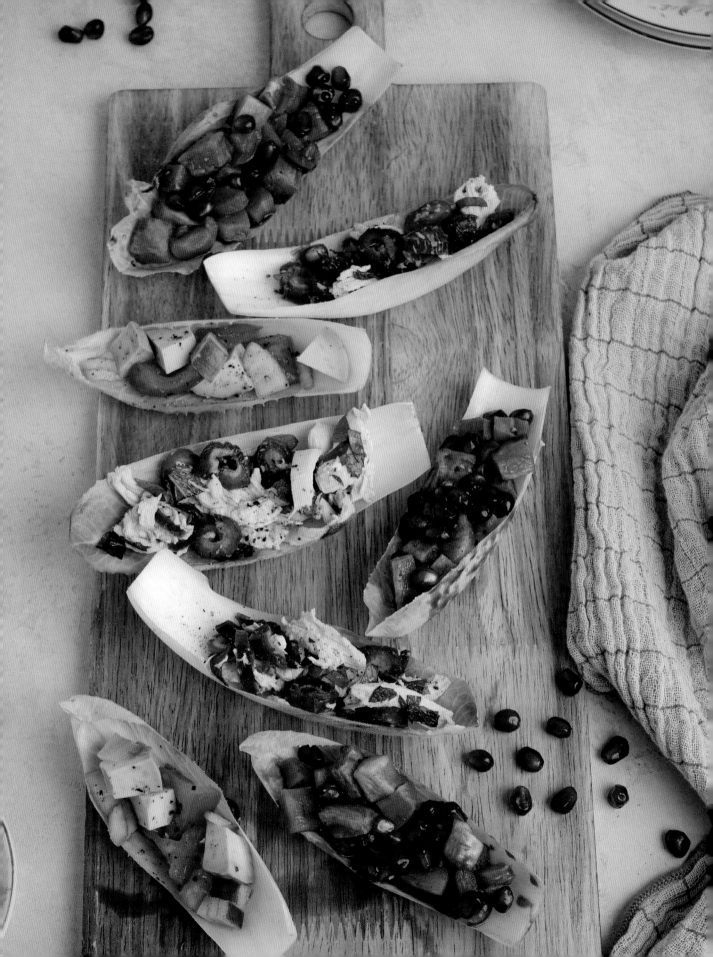

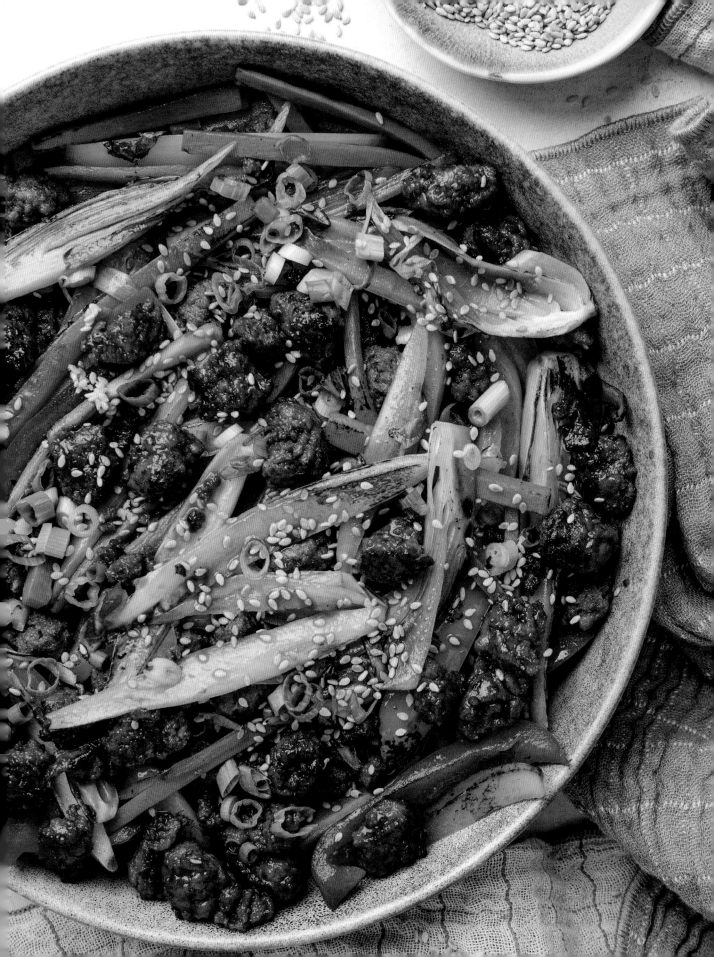

ENDIVE STIR-FRY
WITH VEGETABLES & GROUND TURKEY

Tom: I love stir-fry. Typically, when I want to empty the fridge, stir-fry is the move I make. Stir-fries taste amazing, they hold up great, and they taste even better the next day for a no-hassle lunch. I have even been known to reheat them and then crack a couple eggs to make a breakfast hash. So if you are already a stir-fry fan, I hope you enjoy this one. If you have not made many, hopefully this introduction gets you hooked like I am.

SERVINGS: 4	PREP TIME: 8 MINUTES	TOTAL TIME: 30 MINUTES

2 tablespoons olive oil, divided
1 pound (450g) ground turkey
2 garlic cloves, minced
1 yellow onion, thinly sliced
2 carrots, julienned
1 red bell pepper, thinly sliced
1 yellow bell pepper, thinly sliced
2 endive heads, thinly sliced
2 tablespoons tamari sauce or
    gluten-free soy sauce
1 tablespoon rice vinegar
1 teaspoon honey or maple syrup
Salt and pepper, to taste

SERVING OPTIONS
Chopped green onions
Toasted sesame seeds

1 Heat one tablespoon of olive oil in a large skillet or wok over medium heat. Add the ground turkey and cook, breaking it up with a spatula, until browned and cooked through, about 8 to 10 minutes. Once cooked, transfer the turkey to a plate and set aside.

2 In the same skillet or wok, add the remaining tablespoon of olive oil. Add the garlic and onion, and cook for 2 to 3 minutes until softened.

3 Add the carrot and bell peppers to the skillet and cook for another 3 to 4 minutes until the vegetables are tender-crisp.

4 Add the sliced endive to the skillet and cook for an additional 2 to 3 minutes until wilted but still slightly crisp.

5 Return the cooked turkey to the skillet with the vegetables. Stir in the tamari sauce, rice vinegar, and honey. Season with salt and pepper to taste.

6 Stir everything together and cook for another 1 to 2 minutes until heated through and well combined.

7 Transfer the endive stir-fry to serving plates or bowls. Garnish with chopped green onions and sesame seeds, if desired.

GRILLED ENDIVE

WITH FIG, APPLE & WALNUT SALAD

Rachael: During this week of pregnancy, your sweet little one is becoming more coordinated with their movements, and you may feel their first kicks! (Don't worry if it takes longer to feel movement though. I personally didn't feel those first kicks with my first until week 23.) To stay on theme with experiencing something for the first time, we made grilled endive with fig, apple, and walnut salad, because we're sure most of you have never grilled your lettuce before! Here's to trying and experiencing new things.

SERVINGS: 4	PREP TIME: 10 MINUTES	TOTAL TIME: 20 MINUTES

4 Belgian endive heads
2 tablespoons olive oil
Salt and pepper, to taste

FOR THE FIG, APPLE, AND WALNUT SALAD
4 fresh figs, quartered
1 green apple, thinly sliced
¼ cup chopped walnuts
2 tablespoons balsamic vinegar
1 tablespoon honey or maple syrup
2 tablespoons extra-virgin olive oil
Salt and pepper, to taste
Fresh thyme leaves, optional

1 Preheat a grill to medium-high heat or place a grill pan over medium-high heat.

2 Cut the endive heads in half lengthwise, leaving the stem intact to hold the leaves together.

3 Brush the cut sides of the endive halves with olive oil and season with salt and pepper.

4 Place the endive halves, cut side down, on the preheated grill. Grill for 3 to 4 minutes or until grill marks form and the endive begins to soften.

5 Flip the endive halves and grill for an additional 3 to 4 minutes on the other side until tender.

6 Remove the endive from the grill and set aside.

7 **Prepare the fig, apple, and walnut salad.** In a large bowl, combine the figs, apple, and walnuts.

8 In a small bowl, whisk together the balsamic vinegar, honey, and extra-virgin olive oil until well combined. Season with salt and pepper to taste.

9 Pour the dressing over the fig, apple, and walnut salad. Toss gently to coat everything evenly with the dressing.

10 Arrange the grilled endive halves on a serving platter or individual plates and then spoon the fig, apple, and walnut salad over the top.

11 Garnish the salad with fresh thyme leaves, if desired.

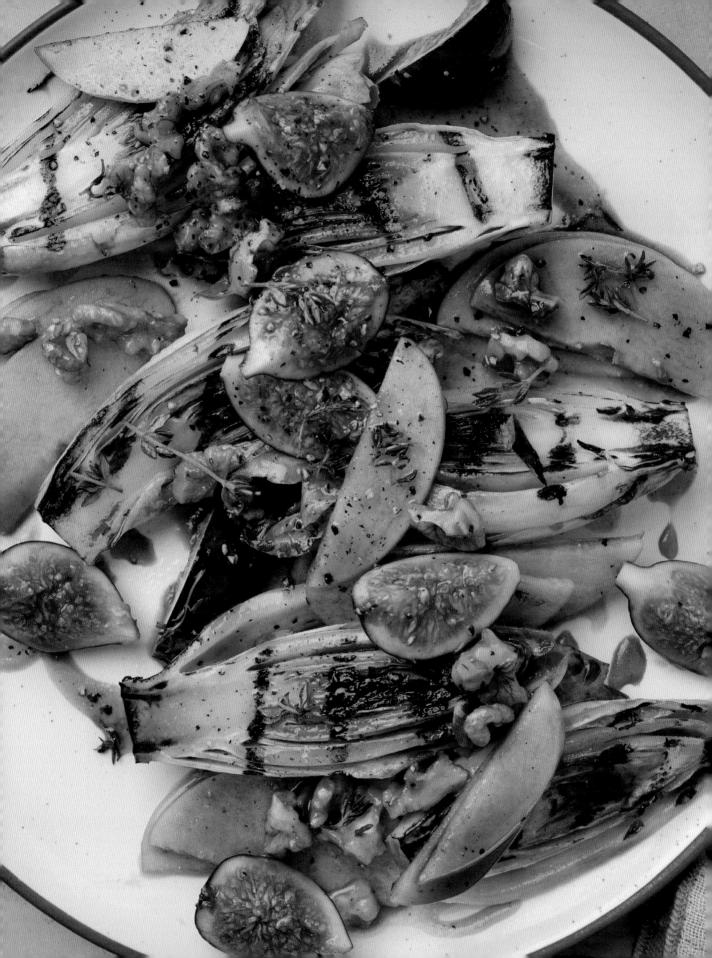

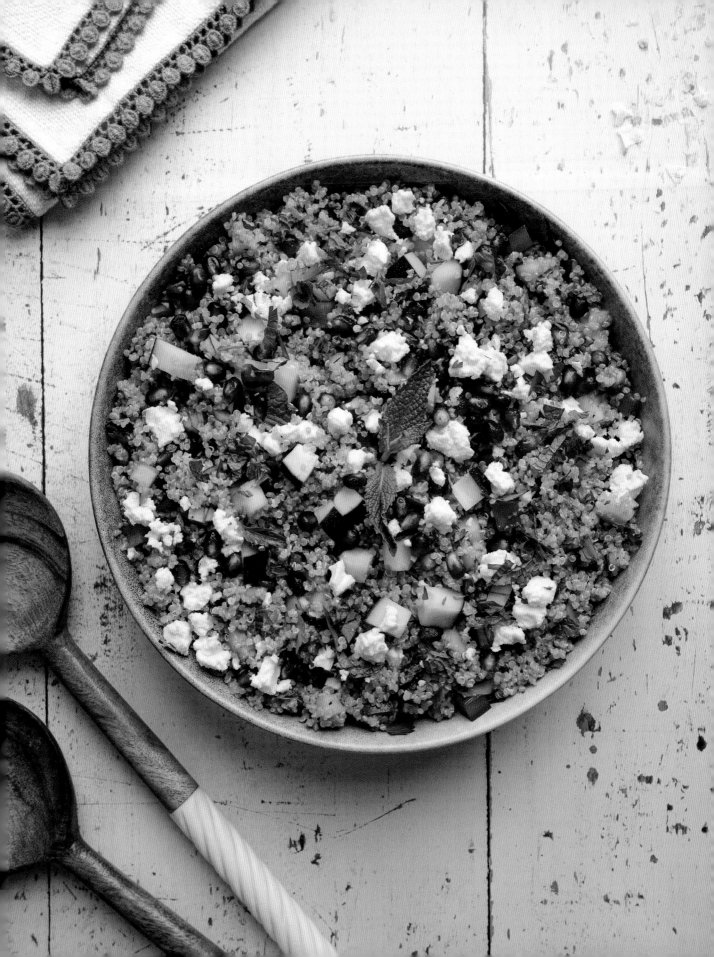

POMEGRANATE QUINOA SALAD

Tom: Let's be honest, quinoa salads are either amazing or extremely bland and boring. As you can imagine, we were not aiming for bland or boring! Start with cooking your quinoa in a flavorful broth and finish with a melody of fresh vegetables, fresh herbs, and the pop of flavor pomegranate brings. This is a flavorful and satisfying dish great for a side or as a light lunch.

SERVINGS: 4	PREP TIME: 10 MINUTES	TOTAL TIME: 30 MINUTES

1 cup white quinoa, rinsed
2 cups vegetable broth or water
½ cup diced cucumber
½ cup diced red bell pepper
¼ cup finely diced red onion
¼ cup chopped fresh parsley
¼ cup chopped fresh mint leaves
½ cup pomegranate arils
¼ cup crumbled feta cheese, optional
¼ cup chopped walnuts, optional

FOR THE DRESSING
Juice and zest of 1 lemon
2 tablespoons extra-virgin olive oil
Salt and pepper, to taste

1 In a medium saucepan, combine the quinoa and vegetable broth with a pinch of salt. Bring to a boil, then reduce the heat to low, cover, and simmer for 15 to 20 minutes or until the quinoa is cooked and the liquid is absorbed. Remove from the heat and let it cool.

2 In a large mixing bowl, combine the cooled quinoa with the cucumber, red bell pepper, red onion, parsley, and mint.

3 Gently fold the pomegranate arils into the salad mixture.

4 **Prepare the dressing.** In a small bowl, whisk together the lemon juice, zest, and extra-virgin olive oil. Season with salt and pepper to taste.

5 Drizzle the dressing over the salad and toss until everything is evenly coated.

6 If desired, sprinkle crumbled feta cheese and chopped walnuts over the salad for added flavor and texture.

7 Serve immediately or refrigerate for a few hours to allow the flavors to meld together.

LEMONADE
WITH POMEGRANATE & ROSEMARY ICE CUBES

Rachael: I love when I get in a "girlhood" mood and do things that are so girlhood coded. Fancy ice cubes scream girlhood to me. It brings me so much cheer to picture a yummy drink with cute ice cubes in an adorable cup! I can name a list of things that will probably stress you out throughout your pregnancy journey, but this simple recipe is intended to bring about joy and cultivate happiness and appreciation for life's simple pleasures.

SERVINGS: 4	PREP TIME: 30 MINUTES	TOTAL TIME: 30 MINUTES, PLUS 4 TO 6 HOURS OR OVERNIGHT TO FREEZE

4 cups water
½ cup honey or maple syrup
Juice of 4–5 large lemons, about 1 cup

FOR THE POMEGRANATE AND ROSEMARY ICE CUBES
1 cup pomegranate juice
Fresh rosemary sprigs

SERVING OPTIONS
Fresh rosemary sprigs
Lemon slices

1 **Prepare the ice cubes.** Pour the pomegranate juice into ice cube trays. Place a small sprig of fresh rosemary into each ice cube compartment, ensuring it is partially submerged in the juice.

2 Place the ice cube trays in the freezer and freeze until solid, about 4 to 6 hours or overnight.

3 **Prepare the lemonade.** In a medium saucepan, add 4 cups of water and gently heat over medium heat.

4 As the water warms, add the honey and stir. This does not need to be at a boil, just warm enough to dissolve the honey. (Adjust the amount of honey to suit your taste.) Once incorporated, allow to cool to room temperature.

5 In a large pitcher, combine the freshly squeezed lemon juice with the honey water. Stir to combine.

6 Once the pomegranate ice cubes are frozen solid, remove them from the ice cube trays and add them to the pitcher of lemonade.

7 Serve the lemonade in glasses making sure to include a pomegranate and rosemary ice cube or two. Optionally, garnish the pitcher or individual glasses with additional rosemary sprigs and lemon slices.

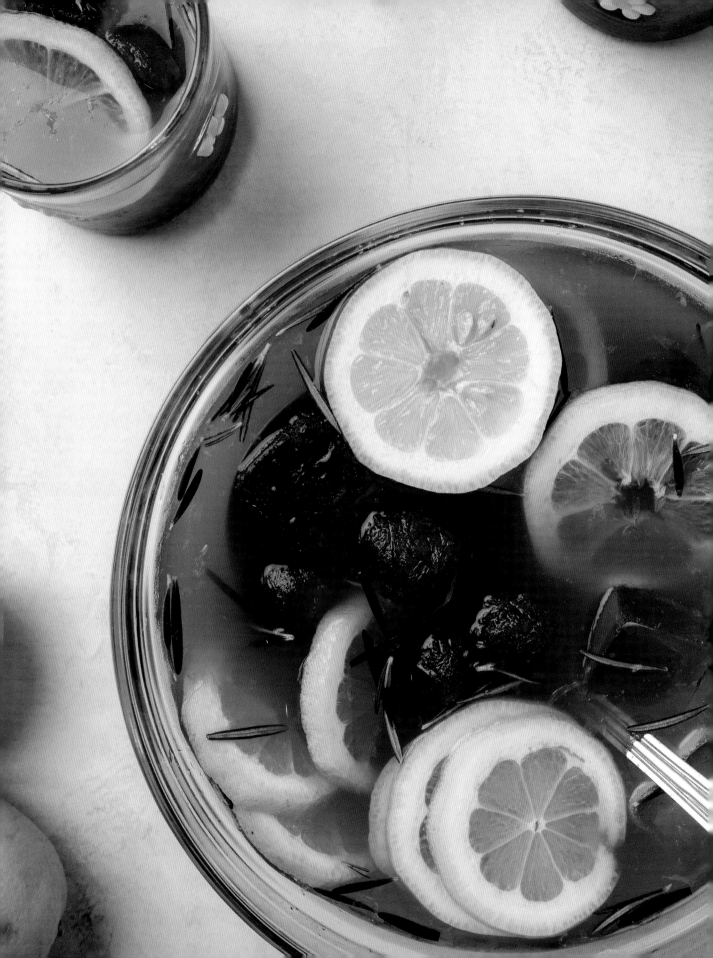

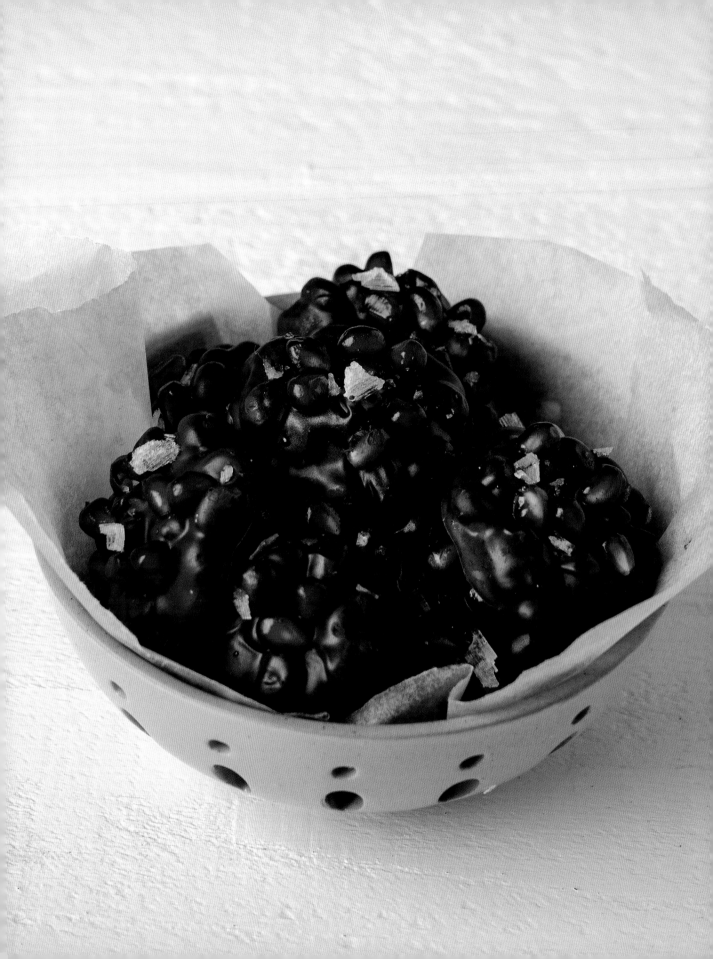

POMEGRANATE & DARK CHOCOLATE BITES

Rachael: Who doesn't have a sweet tooth at some point during their pregnancy? Chocolate and fruit might be one of my favorite dessert combinations. I grew up on chocolate-covered strawberries and the obsession evolved from there. Pomegranate has a literal burst of flavor when you bite into it, so it pairs well with the bitterness of dark chocolate. If you think they look too pretty to eat, it's because it's true—they are beautiful—but please indulge!

SERVINGS: 2	PREP TIME: 10 MINUTES	TOTAL TIME: 40 MINUTES

1 cup dark chocolate chips or chopped dark chocolate, at least 70% cocoa
½ cup pomegranate arils
Flaky sea salt, for optional garnish

1 Place the dark chocolate chips in a microwave-safe bowl. Microwave in 30-second intervals, stirring in between, until the chocolate is completely melted and smooth. Alternatively, you can melt the chocolate using a double boiler on the stovetop.

2 Once the chocolate is melted, gently fold in the pomegranate arils until they are evenly distributed throughout.

3 Line a baking sheet with parchment paper or a silicone baking mat. Using a spoon or a small cookie scoop, drop small dollops of the chocolate and pomegranate mixture onto the prepared baking sheet, spacing them evenly apart.

4 If desired, sprinkle a small pinch of flaky sea salt over each chocolate bite for a sweet-and-salty flavor contrast.

5 Place the baking sheet in the fridge for about 30 minutes or until the chocolate bites are firm and set.

6 Once the chocolate bites are set, remove them from the fridge and serve.

— week 18 —

POMEGRANATE-STUFFED SWEET POTATOES

Rachael: Your anatomy scan should be any day now, if you haven't done it already! I always love being able to spend part of the day seeing our baby. This appointment is meant to take important measurements and make sure everything is progressing as it should, but there is still a nerve-wracking element that comes with it. The nerves you feel will never go away, because you're a parent now and worrying is a part of the job description. To remind you of all the sweetness that still fills this moment, we are serving up a pomegranate-stuffed sweet potato this week. I like to think of it as a healthy savory dessert for dinner that still adds nutritional value to my day.

SERVINGS: 2	**PREP TIME:** 5 MINUTES	**TOTAL TIME:** 1 HOUR

2 medium sweet potatoes
½ cup pomegranate arils
¼ cup chopped pecans or walnuts
2 tablespoons maple syrup or honey
1 tablespoon coconut oil, melted
½ teaspoon ground cinnamon
Pinch of salt

SERVING OPTIONS
Greek yogurt or coconut yogurt
Maple syrup or honey
Chopped fresh parsley

1 Preheat the oven to 400°F (200°C).

2 Wash the sweet potatoes thoroughly and pat them dry with a paper towel. Pierce each sweet potato several times with a fork or knife to allow steam to escape during baking.

3 Place the sweet potatoes on a baking sheet lined with parchment paper or aluminum foil. Bake for 45 to 60 minutes or until the sweet potatoes are tender and can be easily pierced with a fork.

4 While the sweet potatoes are baking, prepare the filling. In a small bowl, combine the pomegranate arils, pecans, maple syrup, melted coconut oil, cinnamon, and a pinch of salt. Mix well to coat everything evenly.

5 Once the sweet potatoes are cooked, remove them from the oven and let them cool slightly. Cut each sweet potato lengthwise down the center, leaving the bottom intact. Gently fluff the flesh with a fork.

6 Divide the pomegranate-and-nut filling evenly among the sweet potatoes, stuffing it into the center of each potato.

7 Serve the stuffed sweet potatoes immediately, topping with a dollop of Greek yogurt, an extra drizzle of maple syrup, and chopped fresh herbs, if desired.

SECOND TRIMESTER
102

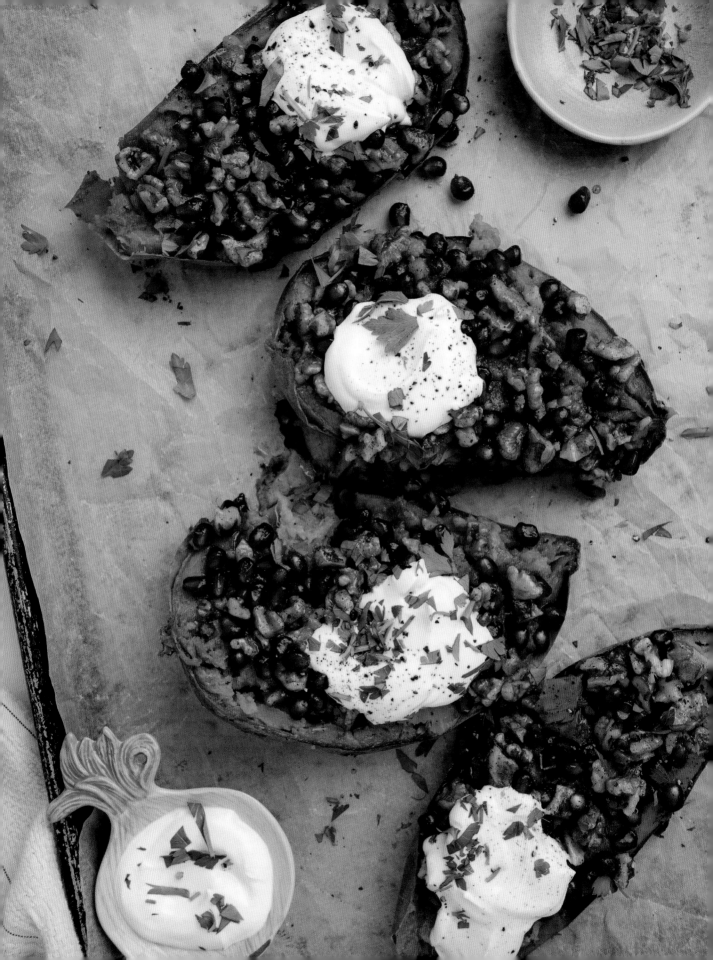

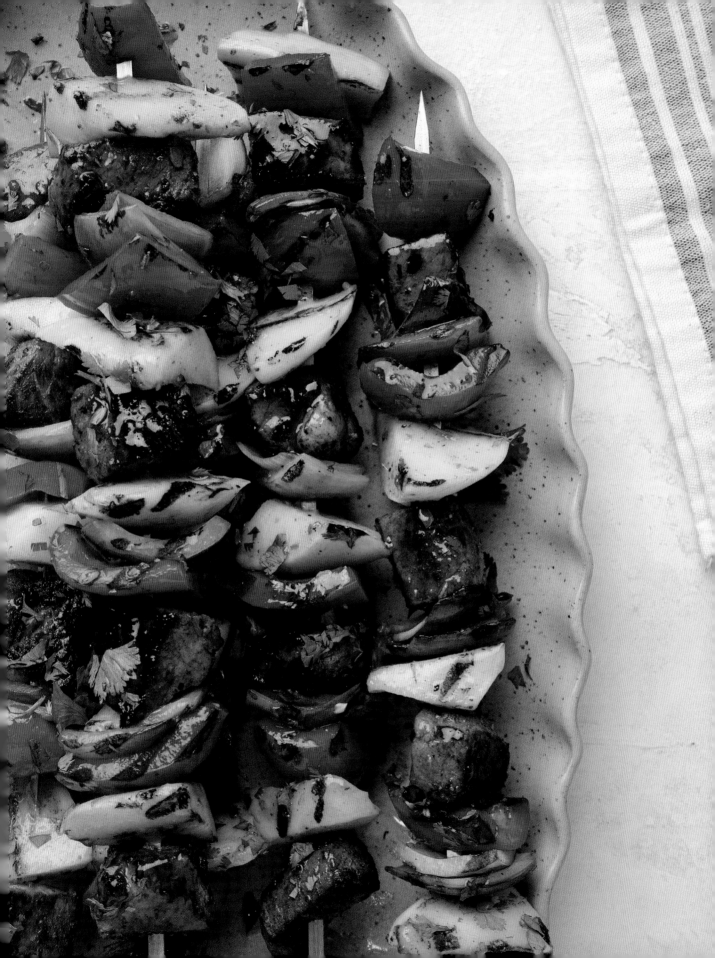

MANGO & BEEF SKEWERS

Tom: Many of these recipes were enjoyed as a family at some sort of celebration. That being said, this recipe is perfect for a party! It is very easy to scale up this recipe to serve a large group. So invite some family and friends over and make some beef, chicken, and veggie skewers, and celebrate your pregnancy journey with loved ones the best way we know how: with food.

SERVINGS: 2–4	PREP TIME: 40 MINUTES	TOTAL TIME: 50 MINUTES, PLUS 30 MINUTES OR OVERNIGHT TO MARINATE

4–8 wooden skewers
3 tablespoons olive oil
3 garlic cloves, minced
1½ teaspoons ground cumin
1½ teaspoons smoked paprika
1 teaspoon salt
½ teaspoon black pepper
1–2 pounds (450-900g) beef sirloin, cut into 1½-inch (3.75cm) cubes
1 ripe mango cut into 1-inch (2.5cm) chunks
1 red bell pepper, cut into 1-inch (2.5cm) chunks
1 red onion, cut into 1-inch (2.5cm) chunks

SERVING OPTIONS
Chopped fresh cilantro
Chopped fresh parsley
Sweet chili dipping sauce

1 Fill a sheet pan or large dish with water and lay your wooden skewers in the water so they begin soaking. Soak the skewers for a minimum of 30 minutes.

2 In a small bowl, combine the olive oil, minced garlic, ground cumin, smoked paprika, salt, and pepper. Add the beef cubes, mango, bell pepper, and onion to the bowl and toss until evenly coated. Let marinate for at least 30 minutes or refrigerate overnight for maximum flavor.

3 Preheat the grill or grill pan over medium-high heat.

4 Thread the marinated beef cubes, mango chunks, red bell pepper chunks, and red onion chunks onto the soaked wooden skewers, until the skewer is filled.

5 Place the assembled skewers on the preheated grill or grill pan. Cook for 3 to 4 minutes on each side or until the beef is cooked to your desired doneness and the vegetables are tender and slightly charred.

6 Remove the skewers from the grill and transfer them to a serving platter.

7 Serve the skewers hot. If desired, garnish with fresh herbs, like cilantro or parsley, and serve with sweet chili sauce for dipping.

Note   *This recipe can also use chicken following the same steps and cooking the chicken 6 to 8 minutes a side or until the internal temperature reaches 165°F (74°C).*

MANGO SMOOTHIE BOWL

Rachael: If there were a list of only 10 dishes I could eat for the rest of my life, a smoothie bowl would be on it. I love customizing each bowl with my favorite fruits, seeds, nuts, nut butters, and quite frankly, anything else I'm feeling that day. For this bowl, instead of topping it with only mangos, we are making a mango-flavored base. If you've been craving cold foods during your pregnancy lately, I'm so happy you landed here. It doesn't matter the season—although, let's be honest, summertime smoothie bowls are superior—these bowls "slap" (which means they always hit the spot).

SERVINGS: 2	**PREP TIME:** 5 MINUTES	**TOTAL TIME:** 10 MINUTES

1 ripe mango, peeled and diced (reserve some for serving)

2 frozen bananas

½ cup plain Greek yogurt or coconut yogurt

¼ cup unsweetened almond milk or coconut milk

1 tablespoon chia seeds or ground flaxseeds

1 tablespoon honey or maple syrup, optional

SERVING OPTIONS

Diced mango

Fresh berries, such as strawberries or blueberries

Granola

Shredded toasted coconut

Chopped nuts or seeds, such as almonds, walnuts, or pumpkin seeds

Fresh mint leaves

1 In a blender, combine the mango, banana slices, Greek yogurt, almond milk, chia seeds, and honey, if using.

2 Blend until smooth and creamy. If the mixture is too thick, you can add more milk to reach your desired consistency.

3 Pour the blended mango smoothie into a bowl.

4 Arrange the diced mango, fresh berries, granola, shredded coconut, and chopped nuts or seeds, and mint leaves on top of the smoothie bowl, as desired.

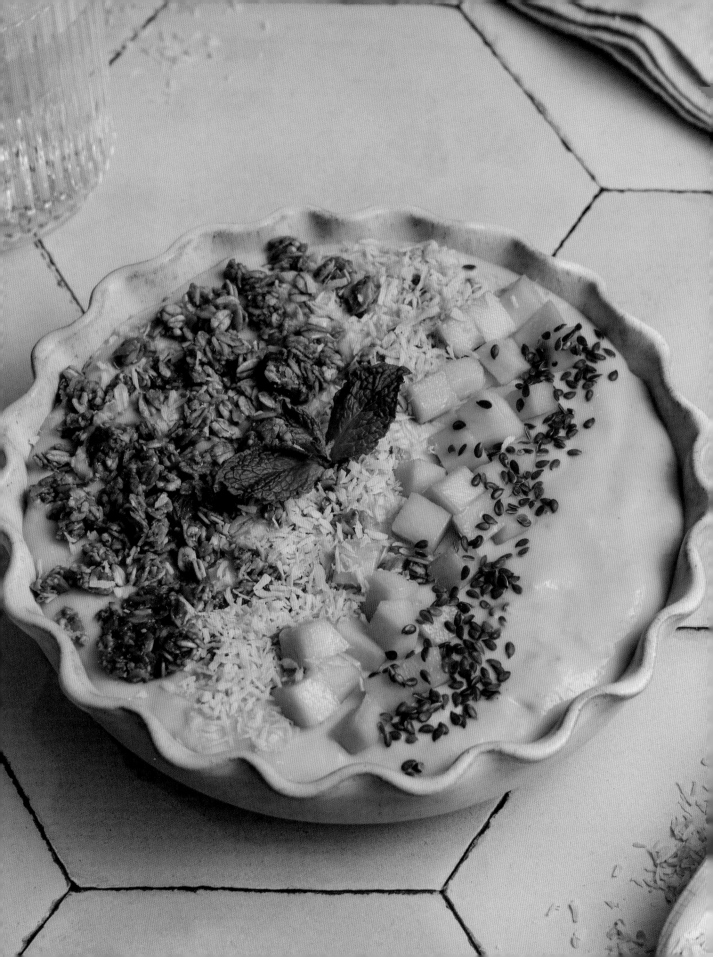

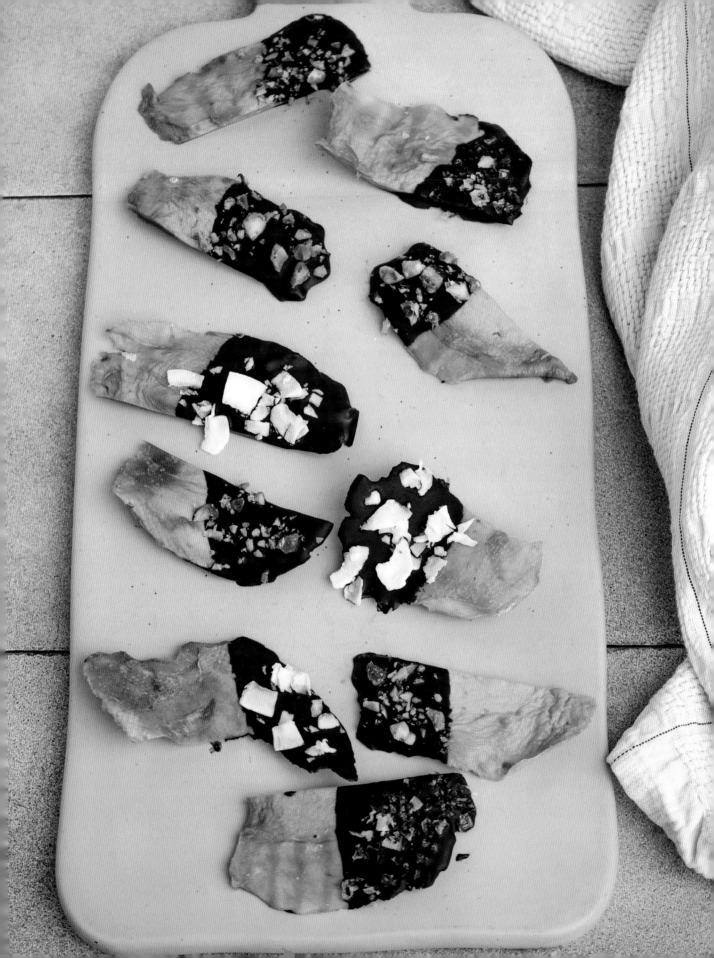

— week 19 —

CHOCOLATE-COVERED DRIED MANGOS

Rachael: When I was going through my fertility journey and learning how to eliminate processed sugars from my diet, I became obsessed with dried mangos. It was my favorite sweet treat because it wasn't full of added sugars but still gave me the sweetness I needed. I told Tom these needed to be included as a recipe in the book, so we gave them a chocolate twist! My hope is that you fall in love with dried mangos as much as I did.

SERVINGS: 1–2	PREP TIME: 8 MINUTES	TOTAL TIME: 30 MINUTES

4 ounces dark chocolate, at least 70% cocoa, chopped
1 tablespoon coconut oil
1 cup dried unsweetened mango slices

SERVING OPTIONS
Sweetened shredded coconut
Chopped pistachio nuts
Flaky sea salt

1 Line a baking sheet with parchment paper or wax paper.

2 In a microwave-safe bowl or double boiler, melt the dark chocolate and coconut oil together until smooth. If using a microwave, heat the chocolate in 30-second intervals, stirring in between, until completely melted.

3 Dip each dried mango slice halfway into the melted chocolate, allowing any excess chocolate to drip off.

4 Place the chocolate-covered mango slices on the prepared baking sheet in a single layer, making sure they are not touching each other.

5 While the chocolate is still melted, sprinkle the chocolate-covered mango slices with shredded coconut, chopped pistachios, or a sprinkle of sea salt flakes, if desired.

6 Place the baking sheet in the fridge for about 15 to 20 minutes or until the chocolate coating has hardened.

DRAGON FRUIT & SHRIMP POKE BOWL
WITH FORBIDDEN BLACK RICE

Rachael: In college, I knew what it was like to be far away from home and crave a home-cooked meal, so one of our favorite ways to give back to our community is to host college meals where students can come over and get free food to go. In the summer of 2024, when I was pregnant with Rosie who was the size of a dragon fruit, we themed the meal around the baby's size and made over 200 of these dragon fruit poke bowls for all the students. Aside from being a delicious take on the poke bowl, I think this is one of the prettiest recipes in the book!

SERVINGS: 4	**PREP TIME:** 25 MINUTES	**TOTAL TIME:** 30 MINUTES

2 tablespoons olive oil

2 garlic cloves, minced

1 tablespoon coconut aminos or tamari

1 tablespoon honey

Juice of 1 lime

Juice of ½ orange

½ teaspoon salt

¼ teaspoon black pepper

1 pound (450g) large shrimp, peeled and deveined, diced into ½-inch (1.25cm) pieces

2 cups cooked black rice (Forbidden)

1 dragon fruit, peeled and diced

1 avocado, sliced

2 tablespoons toasted sesame seeds

¼ cup chopped fresh cilantro

FOR THE POKE SAUCE

2 tablespoons soy sauce or tamari

1 tablespoon rice vinegar

1 tablespoon sesame oil

1 teaspoon honey

1 tablespoon orange juice

1 teaspoon grated fresh ginger

1 teaspoon minced fresh garlic

1 In a medium bowl, whisk together the olive oil, 2 cloves minced garlic, coconut aminos, honey, lime juice, orange juice, salt, and pepper. Add the diced shrimp to the bowl and toss until evenly coated. Let shrimp marinate for at least 15 minutes.

2 Heat a large skillet over medium-high heat. Add the marinated shrimp and sauté for 4 to 5 minutes, until pink and cooked through, stirring often to cook evenly. Remove from heat and set aside.

3 **Prepare the poke sauce.** In a small bowl, whisk together all the sauce ingredients. Set aside.

4 Assemble the poke bowl. Divide the cooked black rice, about ½ cup each, among four bowls, or for presentation, use the hollowed-out dragon fruit skin as two of the bowls. Evenly arrange the cooked shrimp, diced dragon fruit, and sliced avocado over the top of the black rice in each bowl.

5 Drizzle the prepared poke sauce over the ingredients in each bowl.

6 Sprinkle sesame seeds and fresh cilantro over the top before serving.

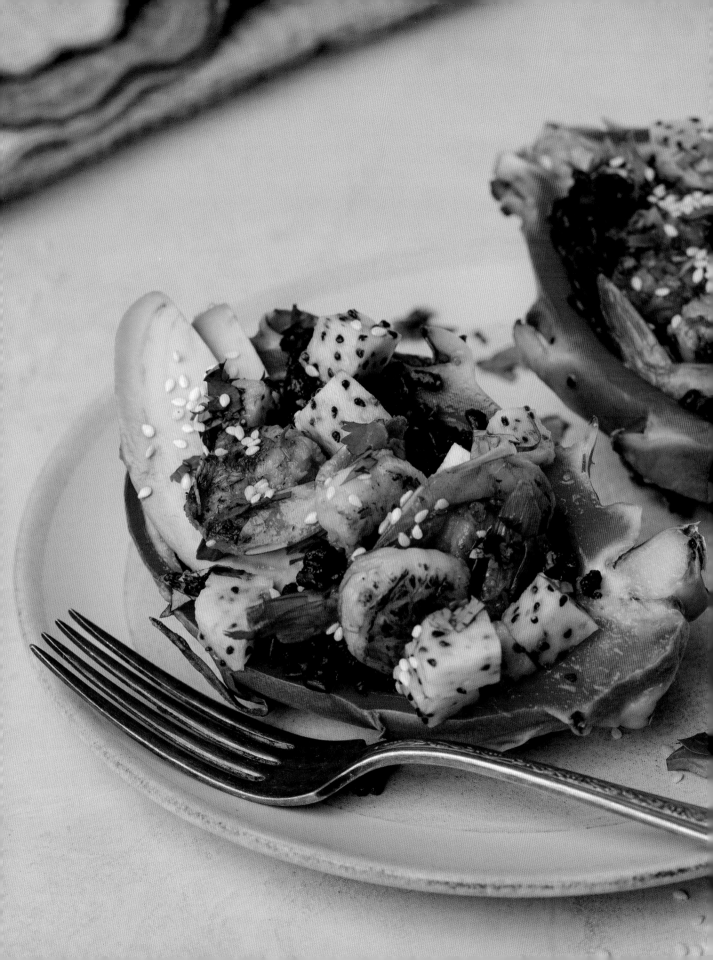

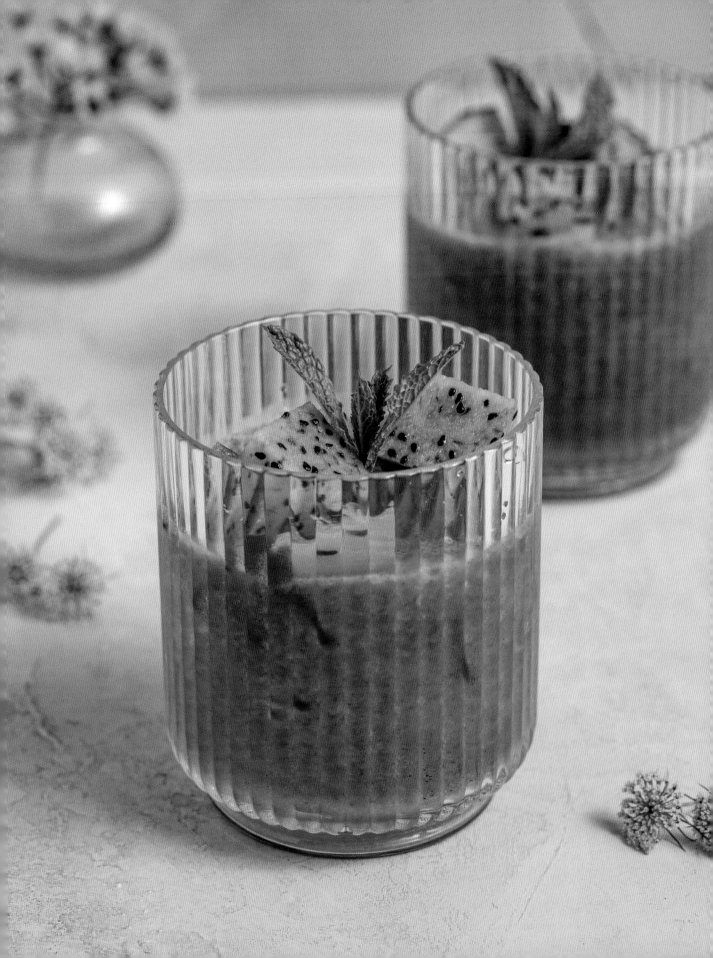

— week 20 —

PINK DRINK

Rachael: Let's take a moment to honor a special milestone of this pregnancy: being at the halfway point! Twenty weeks down with twenty to go (unless baby decides to arrive early). This is a special time to document with photos, if you haven't already. The photos don't have to be fancy either. I love taking just a few Polaroids as a keepsake to look back on one day. We are also going to help you celebrate this week with a fun drink! I love being able to give cheers for milestones, and this drink is a way to do that. And frozen dragon-fruit cubes? Yes, please.

SERVINGS: 2	PREP TIME: 45 MINUTES	TOTAL TIME: 50 MINUTES

1 ripe dragon fruit, peeled and cubed, divided
1 cup fresh strawberries, rinsed and hulled
2 cups canned coconut milk or coconut cream
1 tablespoon lime juice
2 tablespoons honey
Fresh mint leaves, optional, for garnish

1 Spread half the cubed dragon fruit on a baking sheet lined with parchment paper. Place the baking sheet in the freezer for 45 to 60 minutes to use as ice cubes later.

2 To a blender, add the remaining cubed dragon fruit and the strawberries. Pour in the coconut milk, and lime juice. Add the honey, starting with 2 tablespoons and adjusting to your taste preference.

3 Blend the mixture until smooth and well combined.

4 Remove the frozen dragon fruit from the freezer, and fill a glass with a few of the dragon fruit cubes.

5 Pour the blended strawberry and dragon fruit mixture over the cubes.

6 Garnish with fresh mint leaves, if desired.

Notes *If you prefer a lighter flavor, you can use water instead of coconut water as the base. Feel free to add a squeeze of lime juice for a citrusy twist.*

DRAGON FRUIT KABOBS

Tom: The day you start grilling fruit, there is no turning back. I remember the first time I grilled fruit, I thought: *Why would I want to dry out this delicious fruit by sticking it on a hot grill?* I quickly learned it did the complete opposite. The natural sugars caramelize, creating a deeper and more concentrated flavor. The heat slightly softens the fruit while giving it a tender and juicy texture. Lastly, you get the added depth of the smokiness from the grill. I don't know if we call this a side dish or a treat—all I know is that it satisfied Rachael's pregnancy sweet tooth many times!

SERVINGS: 4–6	**PREP TIME:** 35 MINUTES	**TOTAL TIME:** 40 MINUTES

3 dragon fruits, peeled and cut into 1-inch (2.5cm) cubes

2 fresh mango, peeled and cut into 1-inch (2.5cm) cubes

3 kiwis, peeled and cut into quarters

2 cups fresh strawberries, rinsed and hulled

2 cups pineapple chunks

Wooden skewers, soaked in water for 30 minutes

Honey or coconut sugar, optional, for serving

Chopped fresh mint leaves, optional, for garnish

1 Preheat a charcoal grill or a broiler to medium-high.

2 Thread the prepared fruit onto soaked wooden skewers, alternating between the different fruits to create colorful kabobs.

3 Place the kabobs on the grill and turn them every 2 minutes until all sides begin lightly browning. If you're using a broiler, place them on a baking sheet and allow to cook for 2 minutes, remove from the oven, turn the kabobs, and place them back in the oven for 2 more minutes.

4 Drizzle with honey and sprinkle chopped mint over top, if desired.

5 Arrange the fruit kabobs on a serving platter or plate and serve.

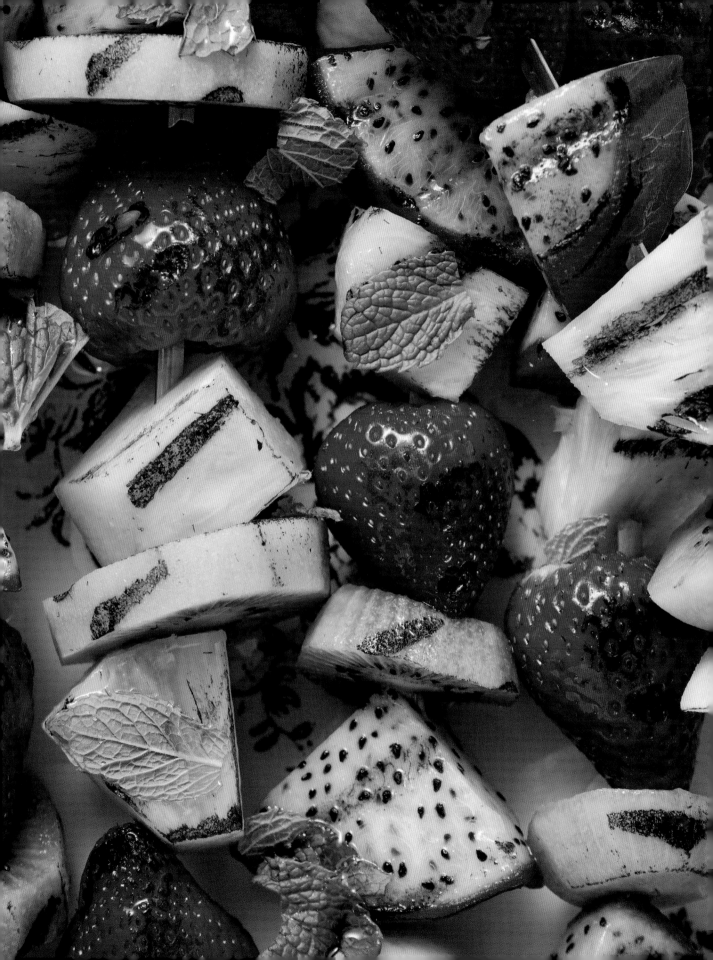

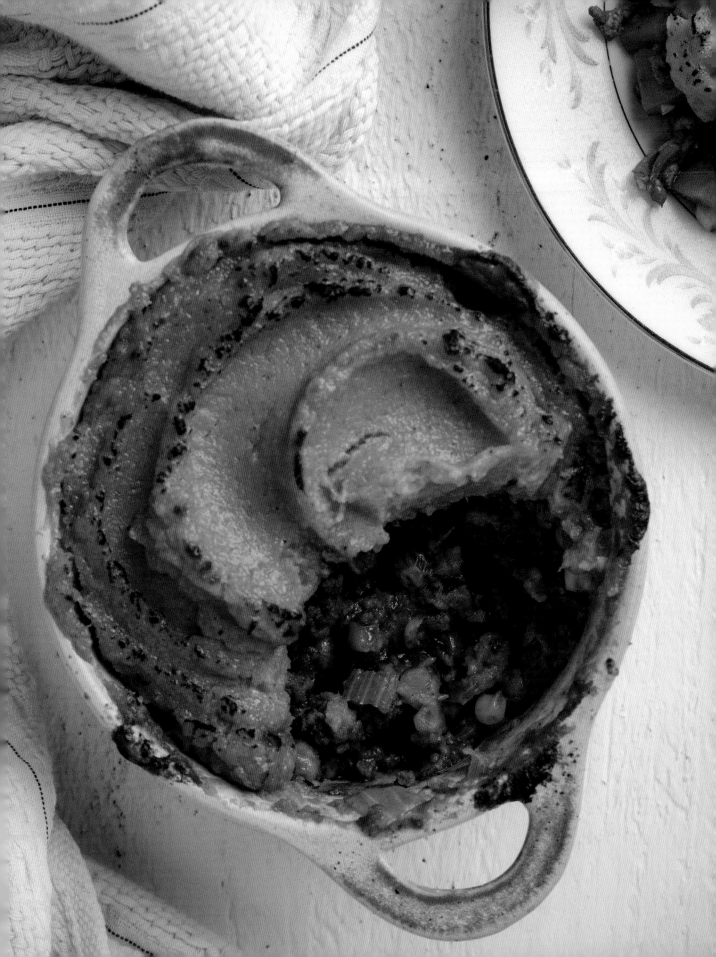

SWEET POTATO SHEPHERD'S PIE

Rachael: A comforting recipe will go a long way during your pregnancy. Once you find your favorites, you will most likely find yourself rotating them into your monthly meal schedule. This shepherd's pie was—and is still—one of my favorite comfort meals. Unlike traditional shepherd's pie made with golden potatoes, this recipe calls for sweet potatoes. This dish will have you reheating leftovers for lunch the next day, if you didn't finish the pan for dinner already.

SERVINGS: 6	PREP TIME: 10 MINUTES	TOTAL TIME: 1 HOUR 25 MINUTES

1 tablespoon olive oil
1 yellow onion, diced
2 garlic cloves, minced
1 pound (450g) ground lamb or ground beef
2 carrots, peeled and diced
2 stalks celery, diced
1 cup peas, fresh or frozen
1 cup corn kernels, fresh or frozen
1 cup beef broth or vegetable broth
2 tablespoons tomato paste
½ tablespoon dried thyme
½ tablespoon dried rosemary
Salt and pepper, to taste

FOR THE SWEET POTATO TOPPING
2 large sweet potatoes, peeled and cubed
2 tablespoons butter or olive oil
¼ teaspoon ground nutmeg
Salt and pepper, to taste

1 **Prepare the sweet potato topping.** Place the cubed sweet potatoes in a large pot and cover with water. Bring to a boil over high heat, then reduce the heat to medium-low and simmer for 15 to 20 minutes or until the sweet potatoes are fork-tender.

2 Drain the sweet potatoes and return them to the pot. Add the butter. Mash the sweet potatoes until smooth and creamy. Season with ground nutmeg, as well as salt and pepper to taste, and set aside.

3 **Make the pie.** Preheat the oven to 375°F (190°C).

4 In a large skillet, heat olive oil over medium heat. Add the onion and garlic, and sauté until softened and fragrant, about 3 to 4 minutes.

5 Add the ground lamb to the skillet and cook until browned, about 7 to 8 minutes, breaking it up as it cooks.

6 Stir in the carrots and celery, and cook for another 5 minutes, until the vegetables start to soften.

7 Add the peas, corn, beef broth, tomato paste, thyme, and rosemary, stir well to combine, and season with salt and pepper to taste. Simmer for 5 to 10 minutes, until the mixture thickens slightly.

8 Transfer the filling mixture to a greased 9x13-inch (23x33cm) baking dish, spreading it out evenly.

9 Spoon the mashed sweet potato topping over the filling, spreading it out with a spatula to cover the entire surface. Use a fork to create ridges on the surface of the sweet potatoes.

10 Place the baking dish in the preheated oven and bake uncovered for 25 to 30 minutes or until the sweet potato topping is lightly golden brown and the filling is bubbly around the edges

11 Remove the shepherd's pie from the oven and let it cool for a few minutes before serving.

SWEET POTATO GNOCCHI
WITH ROASTED ONION & COCONUT SAUCE

Rachael: You are out here making this baby from scratch. Those little fingers, eyes, nose, and that head of hair are the work of you and your amazing body. So making sweet potato gnocchi should be a walk in the park . . . comparatively. Tom paired this gnocchi dish with a roasted onion and coconut sauce. He would say this dish is a celebration of simplicity and depth. I would say it's a badass tutorial to show off that you can do it all: make pasta and make babies from scratch.

SERVINGS: 4	PREP TIME: 25 MINUTES	TOTAL TIME: 1 HOUR 40 MINUTES

2 medium sweet potatoes, about
  1 pound (450g), scrubbed
2 yellow onions
2 tablespoons olive oil, plus more for
  garnish
½ cup full-fat coconut milk
1 tablespoon lemon juice
1 teaspoon salt, divided
¾ cup rice flour (or gluten-free
  all-purpose flour blend), plus more for
  dusting
½ cup potato starch
½ teaspoon ground nutmeg
¼ cup fresh sage leaves, optional

1 Preheat the oven to 400°F (200°C). Line a baking sheet with parchment paper.

2 Prick the sweet potatoes a few times with a fork and place them on the prepared baking sheet. Coat the whole onions lightly with olive oil and place on the baking sheet with the potatoes. Roast the sweet potatoes and onions for about 45 to 60 minutes or until they are fork-tender. Remove the potatoes and onions from the oven and let them cool slightly.

3 Once cooled, cut off the roots and peel the onions, then add them to a blender. Blend on high until very smooth, about 3 minutes. Add the coconut milk and lemon juice and pulse 3 to 4 times to combine. Add ½ teaspoon salt. Taste and adjust seasoning, if needed. Transfer the sauce to a saucepan and keep warm for serving later.

4 Once the sweet potatoes are cool enough to handle, scoop out the flesh and place it in a medium bowl. Mash until smooth.

5 Add the rice flour, potato starch, remaining ½ teaspoon of salt, and ground nutmeg to the mashed sweet potatoes. Mix until a dough forms. If the dough is too sticky, add a little more flour until it becomes easier to handle.

6 Dust a clean surface with rice flour. Divide the dough into 3 smaller portions.

7 Roll each portion of dough into a long rope, about ½ inch (1.25cm) in diameter.

8 Use a knife to cut the rope into small pieces, each about ¾ inch (2cm) in length. You can leave them as is or roll them over a fork to create ridges.

9 Bring a large pot of salted water to a boil. Drop the gnocchi into the boiling water in batches, making sure not to overcrowd the pot.

10 Cook the gnocchi for about 2 to 3 minutes or until they float to the surface. Once they float, let them cook for an additional 1 to 2 minutes.

11 Use a slotted spoon to transfer the cooked gnocchi to a plate or colander. Repeat the steps with the remaining gnocchi.

12 Transfer the cooked gnocchi to a serving plate. Pour the onion sauce on the bottom of the plate around the gnocchi.

13 For an optional garnish, heat a small amount of olive oil in a skillet over medium heat. Once hot, add the sage leaves and fry for about 45 seconds on each side until crispy. Transfer the sage leaves to a wire rack to cool. Garnish each serving of gnocchi with a few of the sage leaves.

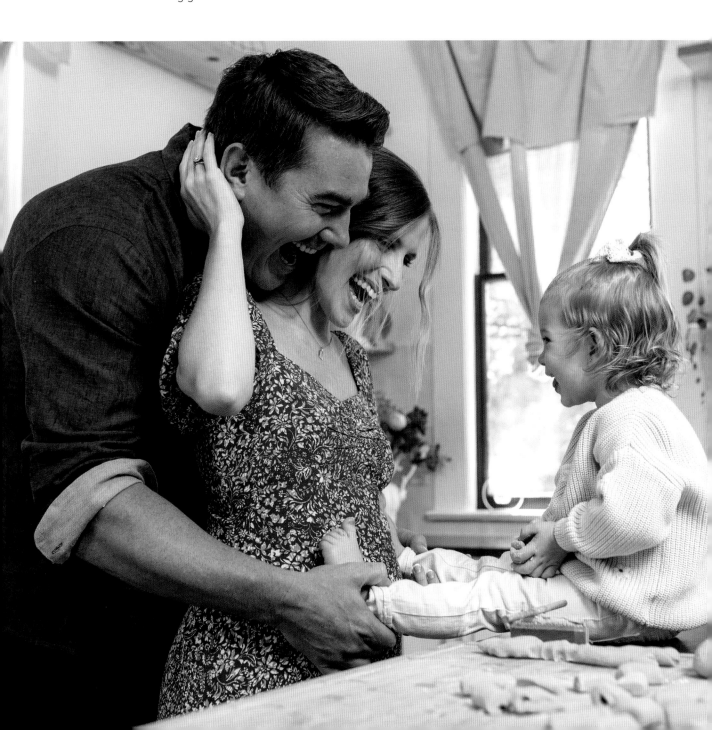

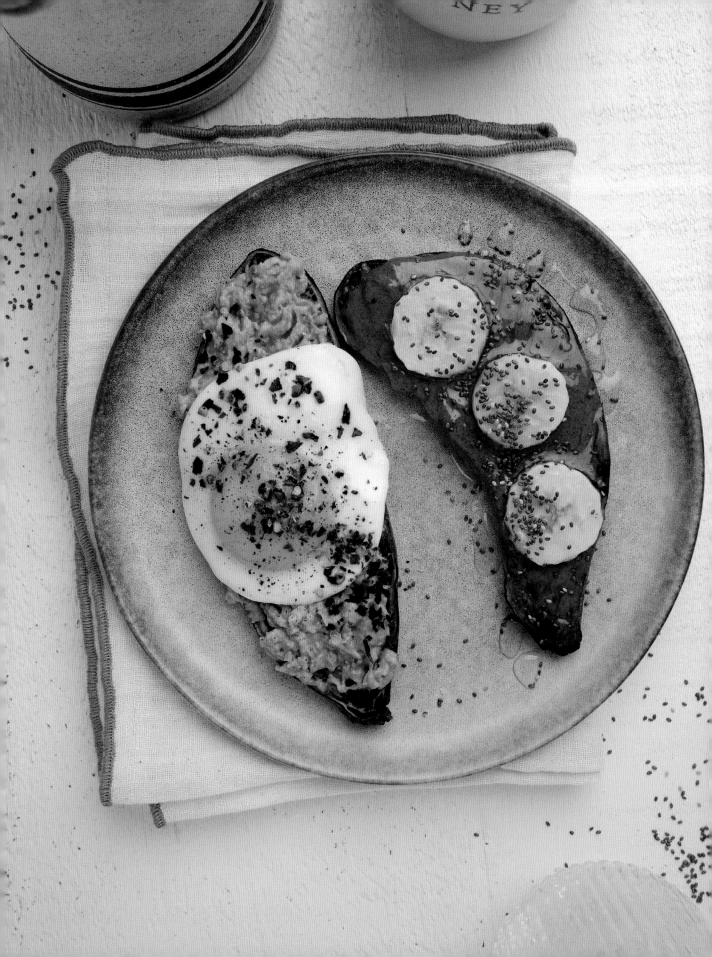

SWEET POTATO TOAST, THREE WAYS

Rachael: I find mornings to be the most intentional time I spend with the baby. Some mornings when I have milestone memories or thoughts about the future, I like to jot them down. It's also the first time of the day to nourish the baby with food, vitamins, and love. Sweet potato toast is a way to get extra nutrients, and it's a switch-up from the typical bread often used.

SERVINGS: 2–4	PREP TIME: 10 MINUTES	TOTAL TIME: 35 MINUTES

1 large sweet potato, washed and sliced lengthwise into ¼-inch thick slices
Olive oil or coconut oil, for brushing
Salt and pepper, to taste

AVOCADO & EGG TOAST
1 ripe avocado, mashed
2 large eggs, cooked to your preference
Red pepper flakes
Fresh herbs, your choice

ALMOND BUTTER & BANANA TOAST
¼ cup almond butter or any nut or seed butte
1 ripe banana, thinly sliced
Chia seeds
Drizzle of honey, optional

SMOKED SALMON & CREAM CHEESE TOAST
4 ounces (113g) smoked salmon
¼ cup cream cheese or dairy-free cream cheese
Capers
Chopped fresh dill

1 Preheat the oven to 400°F (200°C).

2 Arrange the sweet potato slices in a single layer on a baking sheet lined with parchment paper.

3 Brush both sides of the sweet potato slices with olive oil and season with salt and pepper, to taste.

4 Bake in the preheated oven for 20 to 25 minutes, flipping halfway through, or bake until the sweet potatoes are tender and lightly browned around the edges.

5 Assemble your choice of toast.

FOR AVOCADO & EGG TOAST

1 Spread mashed avocado onto each sweet potato slice. Top with your choice of cooked eggs (poached, scrambled, or fried) and sprinkle with red pepper flakes, fresh herbs, and additional salt and pepper, to taste.

2 Arrange the prepared sweet potato toasts on a serving platter and serve.

FOR ALMOND BUTTER & BANANA TOAST

1 Spread almond butter onto each sweet potato slice. Arrange banana slices on top and sprinkle with chia seeds. Drizzle with honey, if desired.

2 Arrange the prepared sweet potato toasts on a serving platter and serve.

FOR SMOKED SALMON & CREAM CHEESE TOAST

1 Spread cream cheese onto each sweet potato slice. Top evenly with smoked salmon and garnish with capers and fresh dill.

2 Arrange the prepared sweet potato toasts on a serving platter and serve.

CANDIED GRAPEFRUIT PARFAIT

Rachael: I had a weird texture thing when it came to yogurt during my pregnancies. During my first pregnancy, even the thought of yogurt made my stomach turn. However, during my second pregnancy, I had a yogurt parfait at least twice a week. It's crazy how each pregnancy can vary. If you are currently loving yogurt, then please enjoy this delicious grapefruit parfait. If yogurt is on your "do not mess with" list, be sure to revisit this recipe after the baby is born!

SERVINGS: 2	PREP TIME: 10 MINUTES	TOTAL TIME: 25 MINUTES

1 large grapefruit
¼ cup honey or maple syrup
¼ cup water
Pinch of salt

FOR THE PARFAITS
1 cup Greek yogurt or dairy-free yogurt
¼ cup granola
¼ cup chopped nuts, such as almonds, pecans, or walnuts
Fresh mint leaves, optional

1. Leaving the peel on, cut the grapefruit into ½ -inch-thick (1.25cm) round slices.

2. In a large skillet, combine the honey, water, and a pinch of salt. Heat over medium heat until the mixture comes to a simmer.

3. Add the quartered grapefruit slices to the skillet in a single layer. Cook for about 5 to 7 minutes on each side, until the grapefruit slices are caramelized and the syrup has thickened slightly. Be careful not to let them burn.

4. Once caramelized, remove the grapefruit slices from the skillet and let them cool on a wire rack or plate.

5. **Assemble the parfaits.** In serving glasses or bowls, layer a ¼ cup Greek yogurt, 1 or 2 candied grapefruit slices, and a sprinkle of granola and chopped nuts. Repeat the layers until the glasses are filled.

6. Garnish the parfaits with fresh mint leaves, if desired, for a pop of color and extra freshness.

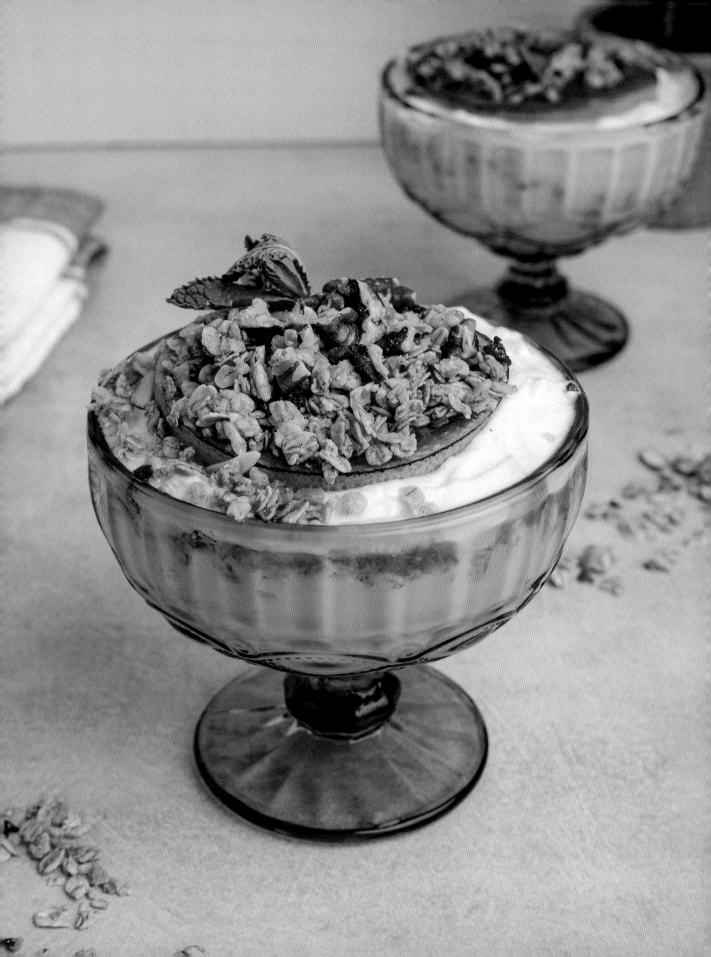

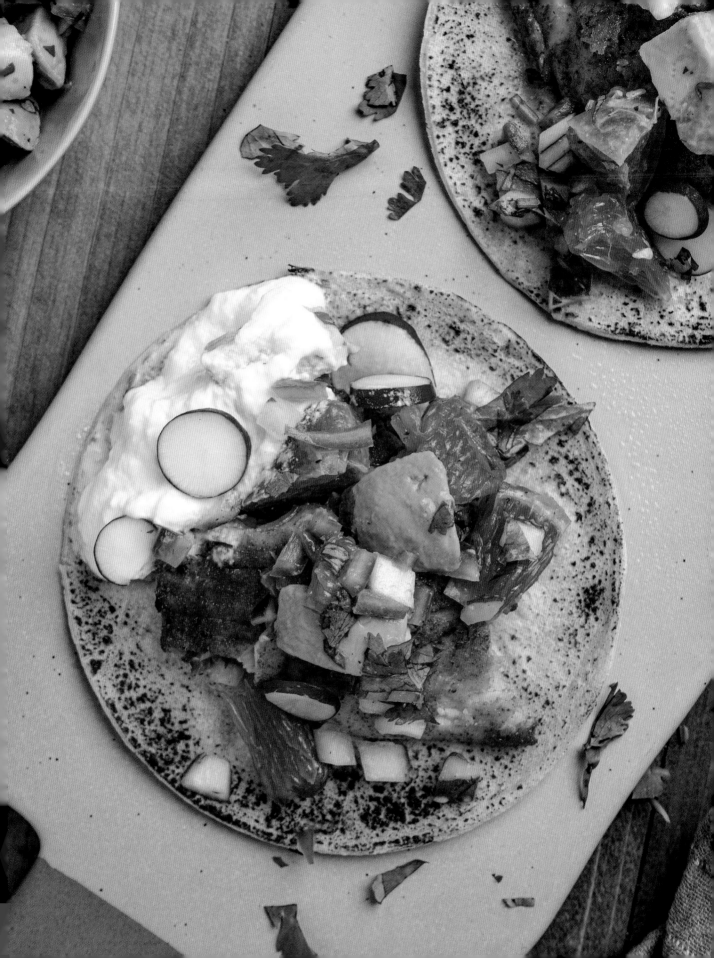

— week 22 —

FISH TACOS

WITH GRAPEFRUIT AVOCADO SALSA

Tom: Salsas are so versatile, as you will take note with this one. Sweet, spicy, chunky, finely chopped, liquefied—salsas can be made in a variety of ways, and that's what I love about them so much. Just like with babies, no two salsas will ever be the same, and each is special in their own way. Served with a protein of choice made into tacos or on their own with a bag of chips, you'll find this salsa to be a refreshing fruit-forward blend of flavors.

SERVINGS: 2–3	**PREP TIME:** 10 MINUTES	**TOTAL TIME:** 20 MINUTES

1 pound (450g) whitefish fillets, such as
   cod or mahi mahi
1 teaspoon ground cumin
1 teaspoon paprika
Salt and pepper, to taste
1 tablespoon olive oil
4-6 corn tortillas

FOR THE SALSA
1 large grapefruit, peeled and
   segmented into ½-inch pieces
1 ripe avocado, diced
¼ cup finely chopped red onion
¼ cup chopped fresh cilantro
1 jalapeño, ribs and seeds removed,
   finely chopped
Juice of 1 lime
Salt and pepper, to taste

SERVING OPTIONS
Shredded cabbage
Sliced radishes
Greek yogurt or sour cream

1 **Prepare the salsa.** In a mixing bowl, combine all the salsa ingredients and toss well until mixed thoroughly. Refrigerate until ready to use.

2 **Make the tacos.** Pat the fish fillets dry with paper towels. Season both sides of the fish with ground cumin, paprika, salt, and pepper.

3 Heat the olive oil in a large skillet over medium-high heat. Once hot, add the seasoned fish fillets to the skillet and cook for 3 to 4 minutes per side or until cooked through and flaky. Remove from heat and set aside.

4 Wrap the corn tortillas in parchment paper and place on a microwave-safe plate. Microwave them for 30 to 40 seconds or until the tortillas are warmed through.

5 Assemble the tacos by adding a few pieces of fish with a generous spoonful of the salsa on top of each of the warmed tortillas.

6 Add any optional toppings such as shredded cabbage, sliced radishes, or a dollop of Greek yogurt before serving.

Notes   *Alternatively, you can serve the grapefruit avocado salsa as a side salad by itself or alongside grilled chicken, shrimp, or any other protein of your choice. Simply spoon the salsa into a serving bowl and garnish with extra cilantro, if desired.*

ROSEMARY GRAPEFRUIT GRANITA

Rachael: At this time, I would like you to play "Ice Ice Baby" by Vanilla Ice, because this week we are celebrating that sweet little baby with shaved ice, or a *granita*, more specifically. Think of this recipe as a DIY snow cone, if you will, but in our opinion: better. Once you master this recipe, don't be surprised if you find yourself trying to use different fruits, like strawberries, watermelon, or lemon to satisfy your sweet treat craving all year long.

SERVINGS: 2	**PREP TIME:** 15 MINUTES	**TOTAL TIME:** 3 HOURS 15 MINUTES

2 large pink grapefruits
½ cup water
¼ cup honey (adjust to taste)
Zest of 1 grapefruit
2 sprigs fresh rosemary, plus more for garnish
Edible flowers, for garnish (optional)

1 After removing the zest from 1 grapefruit, cut the grapefruits in half and juice them to yield approximately 1½ cups of grapefruit juice. Strain the juice to remove any pulp and seeds.

2 In a small saucepan, combine the water, honey, fresh rosemary sprigs, and grapefruit zest.

3 Bring the mixture to a simmer over medium heat, stirring occasionally, until the honey has dissolved and the mixture is fragrant, about 5 minutes.

4 Remove the saucepan from heat and let the rosemary steep in the syrup as it cools to room temperature.

5 Once the rosemary syrup has cooled, strain it through a fine-mesh sieve to remove the rosemary sprigs and grapefruit zest.

6 In a large bowl, mix the strained rosemary syrup and grapefruit juice. Taste and adjust sweetness, if needed, by adding more honey.

7 Pour the grapefruit and rosemary syrup mixture into a 9x13-inch (23x33cm) freezerproof baking dish (metal freezes best). Place the dish in the freezer and let it freeze for about 1 hour.

8 After 1 hour, use a fork to scrape and stir the partially frozen mixture, breaking up any large ice crystals.

9 Return the dish to the freezer and continue to scrape and stir every 30 minutes to 1 hour, until the granita is completely frozen and has a fluffy, icy texture, about 3 hours.

10 Once the granita is fully frozen, use a fork to scrape it into fluffy ice crystals. Spoon the granita into serving dishes or glasses. Garnish with edible flowers or fresh rosemary sprigs, if desired.

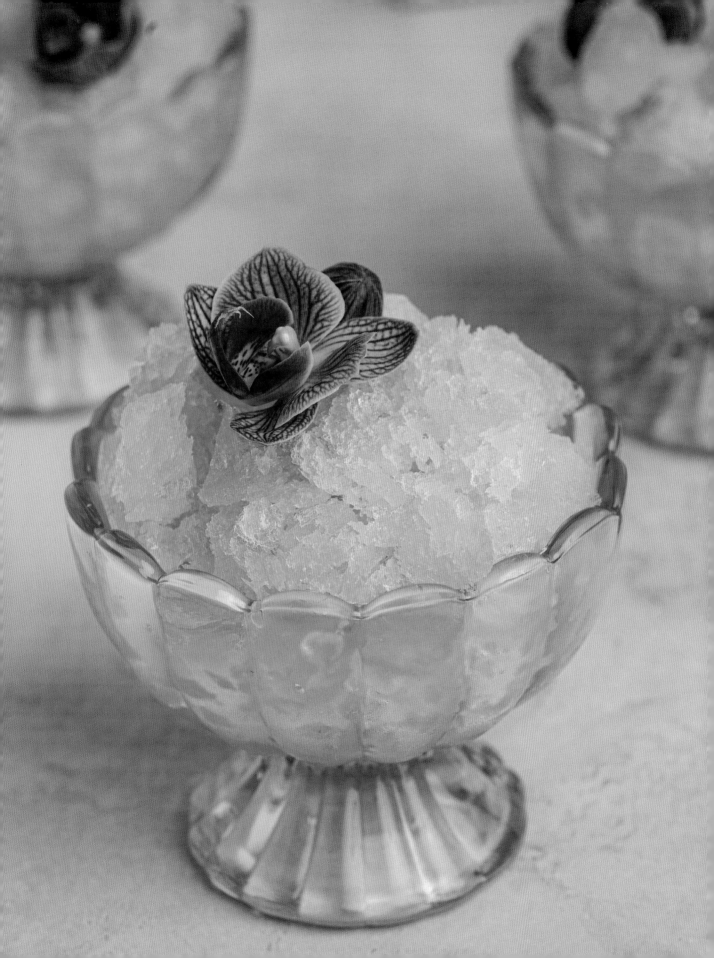

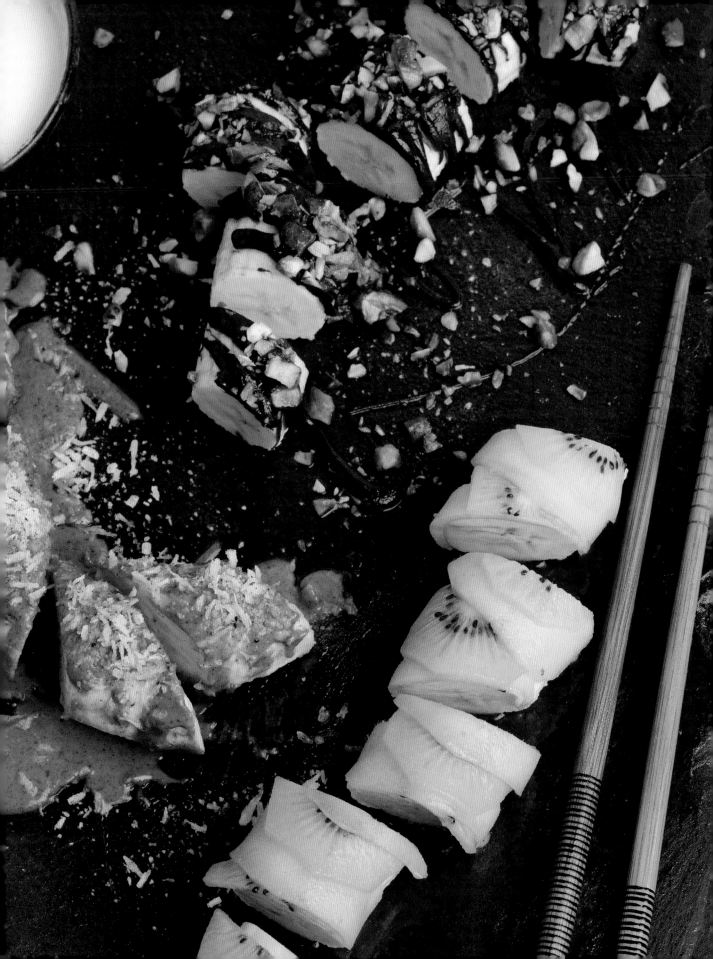

BANANA SUSHI, THREE WAYS

Rachael: Welcome to your fruit-sushi making class at home! We absolutely love this recipe because it's simply just fun. The first time Tom made this banana sushi, I was so impressed with how it turned out and how realistic some of the "rolls" looked. And because you can never order just one roll when you order sushi, we made sure to cover all the bases and include a chocolate, an almond butter, and a fruit-covered option. Whether it's date night or a fun activity to do with your kids, these will be a fun memory to make.

SERVINGS: 3	PREP TIME: 10 MINUTES	TOTAL TIME: 15 MINUTES

CHOCOLATE & PISTACHIO BANANA SUSHI

3 firm bananas

½ cup semisweet morsels (we like Enjoy Life Foods)

⅓ cup crushed pistachios

Plain cashew yogurt or Greek yogurt

ALMOND BUTTER & COCONUT BANANA SUSHI

3 firm bananas

⅓ cup almond butter

⅓ cup toasted coconut flakes

Plain cashew yogurt or Greek yogurt

KIWI-MANGO-BANANA SUSHI

3 firm bananas

1 mango

2 kiwis

¼ cup honey

Plain cashew yogurt or Greek yogurt

FOR CHOCOLATE & PISTACHIO BANANA SUSHI

1 Peel the bananas, leaving the fruit whole, and place them on a serving plate.

2 Melt the chocolate using a double boiler or by placing it in a microwave-safe bowl and microwaving for 30-second intervals, stirring after each interval, until melted.

3 Drizzle the melted chocolate over the bananas and then sprinkle with the crushed pistachios.

4 Slice the bananas into ½-inch (1.25cm) coins. Using chopsticks, dip the bananas into your favorite yogurt and enjoy.

FOR ALMOND BUTTER & COCONUT BANANA SUSHI

1 Peel the bananas, leaving the fruit whole, and place them on a serving plate.

2 Spread the desired amount of almond butter on the bananas and then sprinkle coconut flakes over top.

3 Slice the bananas into ½-inch (1.25cm) coins. Using chopsticks, dip the bananas into your favorite yogurt and enjoy.

FOR KIWI-MANGO-BANANA SUSHI

1 Peel the bananas, leaving the fruit whole, and place them on a serving plate.

2 Peel and thinly slice the mango and kiwis.

3 Pour the honey over the bananas and layer by alternating slices of the kiwi and mango overlapping slightly.

4 Slice the bananas into ½-inch (1.25cm) coins. Using chopsticks, dip the bananas into your favorite yogurt.

BANANA FRENCH TOAST

Rachael: We're bringing it back to the basics with a classic banana French toast. As a noncook who helped edit and formulate the recipes each week, I wanted Tom to include some of our favorite basic recipes that always hit home, and there's nothing I love more than a slow morning with French toast, bacon, a glass of orange juice, and the word scramble section of the newspaper. I have a sneaky suspicion that the baby will love this recipe too.

SERVINGS: 2–4	PREP TIME: 5 MINUTES	TOTAL TIME: 15 MINUTES

2 ripe bananas

2 large eggs

¼ cup unsweetened almond milk or coconut milk

1 teaspoon vanilla extract

½ teaspoon ground cinnamon

4 slices gluten-free bread of choice

2 tablespoons coconut oil or ghee

SERVING OPTIONS

Sliced bananas

Fresh berries

Maple syrup

Nut butters

Powdered sugar

Whipped cream (we like coconut whip)

1 In a shallow bowl that is large enough to fit your bread, mash the ripe bananas with a fork until smooth.

2 Add the eggs, almond milk, vanilla extract, and ground cinnamon to the mashed bananas. Whisk until well combined.

3 Soak each slice of bread into the banana mixture for a few seconds, making sure to coat both sides evenly.

4 Heat a large skillet or frying pan over medium heat. Add a small amount of coconut oil to coat the pan.

5 Place the soaked bread slices in the pan and cook for 2 to 3 minutes on each side or until golden brown and cooked through.

6 Once cooked, cut the French toast in half on the diagonal and serve with your choice of toppings, such as sliced bananas, fresh berries, maple syrup, or nut butter.

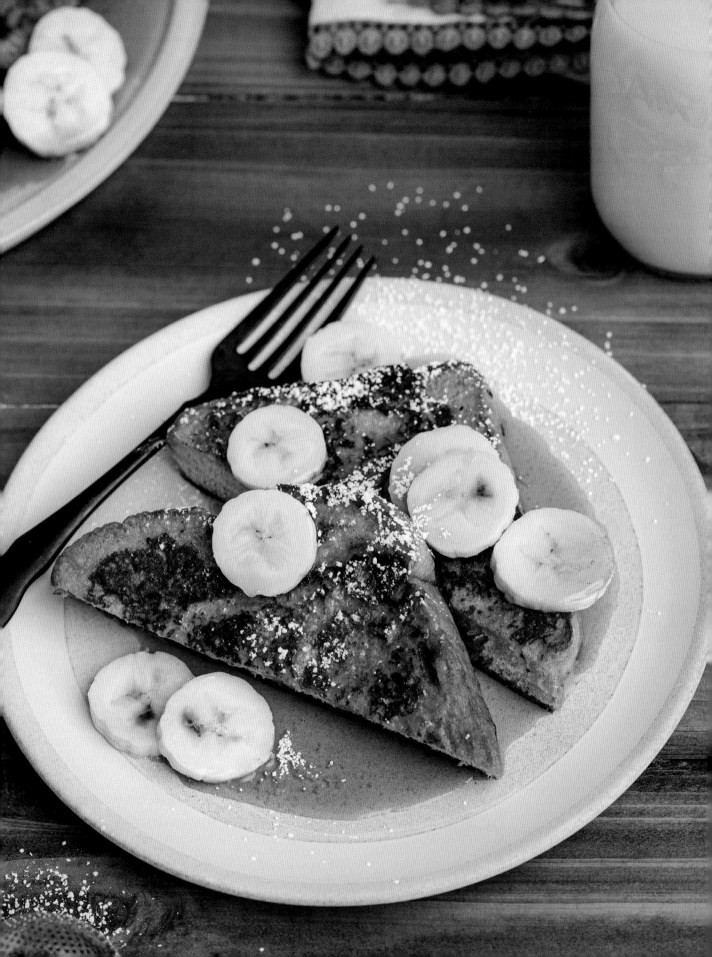

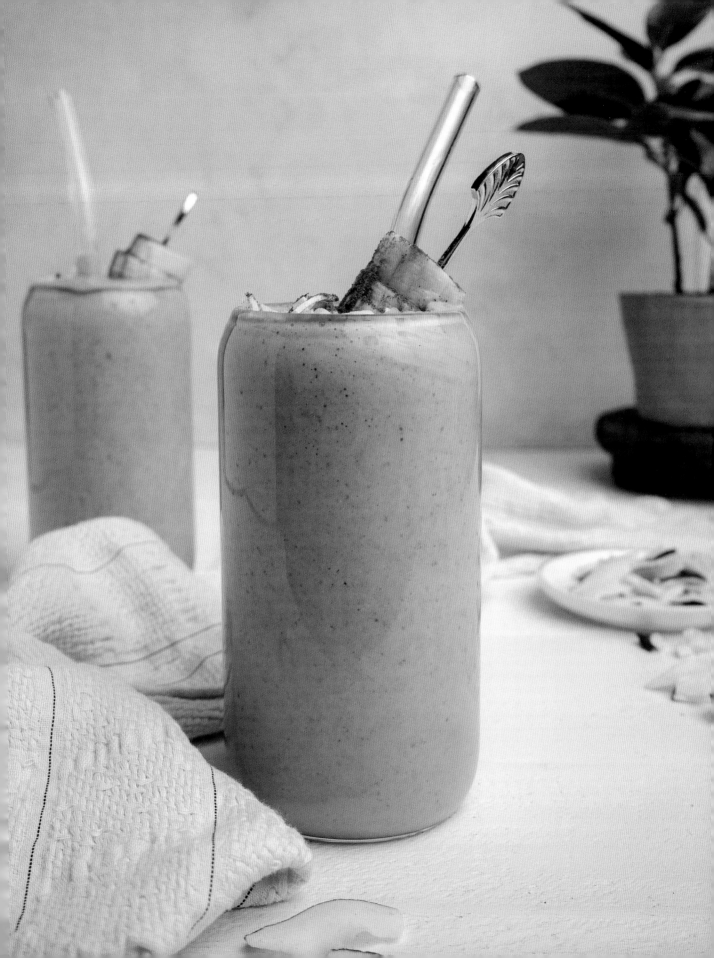

BANANA RECOVERY SMOOTHIE

Rachael: I kid you not, I drank this smoothie every day during the second trimester of my pregnancy. This recipe is inspired by a café I would visit in Raleigh, North Carolina, that sold a smoothie with these ingredients. At 8 a.m., when the café opened, I had this drink on auto order, and it was made and delivered to our house every morning. When I realized how much money we were spending on smoothies each week, we learned how to make a rendition of it at home. Without further ado, your new staple smoothie is here.

SERVINGS: 2–4	**PREP TIME:** 5 MINUTES	**TOTAL TIME:** 15 MINUTES

2 bananas, frozen
1 cup frozen cherries
¼ cup cashews
1 scoop vegan protein powder
1 tablespoon honey
1 cup almond milk
3 ice cubes
½ cup coconut yogurt

SERVING OPTIONS
Sliced bananas
Unsweetened shredded coconut
Sprinkle of ground cinnamon

1 Add bananas, cherries, cashews, protein powder, honey, almond milk, ice cubes, and yogurt to a blender. Add the yogurt last so it doesn't stick to the bottom of the blender.

2 Blend on high speed until smooth and creamy. Add more ice cubes or almond milk to adjust the consistency to your liking.

3 Pour the smoothie into glasses and garnish with optional toppings such as sliced banana, shredded coconut, or a sprinkle of cinnamon.

CARROT RIBBON SALAD

Tom: Just a friendly reminder that nobody's perfect. Despite checking the photos and recipes countless times, somehow this one slipped through the cracks. As you'll notice, the picture is missing chickpeas and cherries. Credit to Rachael for questioning me about this recipe, yet somehow it still managed to slip by. I love this recipe so much that it was the first one featured on our website. It is refreshing, loaded with nutrients, and has become a lunchtime staple for us. Whether you're expecting your first baby or adding to your family, let's celebrate another week together. Imperfections and all, let's rejoice in the fact that we don't have to be flawless.

SERVINGS: 4	PREP TIME: 15 MINUTES	TOTAL TIME: 30 MINUTES

4 large carrots, peeled
¼ cup chopped fresh parsley
2 tablespoons chopped walnuts or cashews
¼ cup dried cherries or cranberries
¼ cup chickpeas, rinsed and drained, optional
1 tablespoon toasted white sesame seeds, optional

FOR THE DRESSING
2 tablespoons extra-virgin olive oil
1 tablespoon apple cider vinegar
1 tablespoon lemon juice
1 teaspoon maple syrup (adjust to taste)
Salt and pepper, to taste

1 Make your carrot ribbons. Using a vegetable peeler or mandoline, thinly slice the length of the carrot to get long ribbons. Place the ribboned carrots in a large mixing bowl.

2 **Prepare the dressing.** In a small bowl, whisk together the dressing ingredients until well combined.

3 Pour the dressing over the thinly sliced carrots in the mixing bowl.

4 Add the parsley to the bowl.

5 Toss everything together until the carrots are evenly coated with the dressing and the parsley is well distributed.

6 Add chopped walnuts, dried cherries, and chickpeas (if using) to the salad for added crunch and protein.

7 Transfer the dressed carrot salad to the refrigerator to chill for 15 to 20 minutes.

8 Remove from the refrigerator when ready to serve. Transfer onto a serving plate. Sprinkle sesame seeds on top for an extra pop of flavor and visual appeal, if desired.

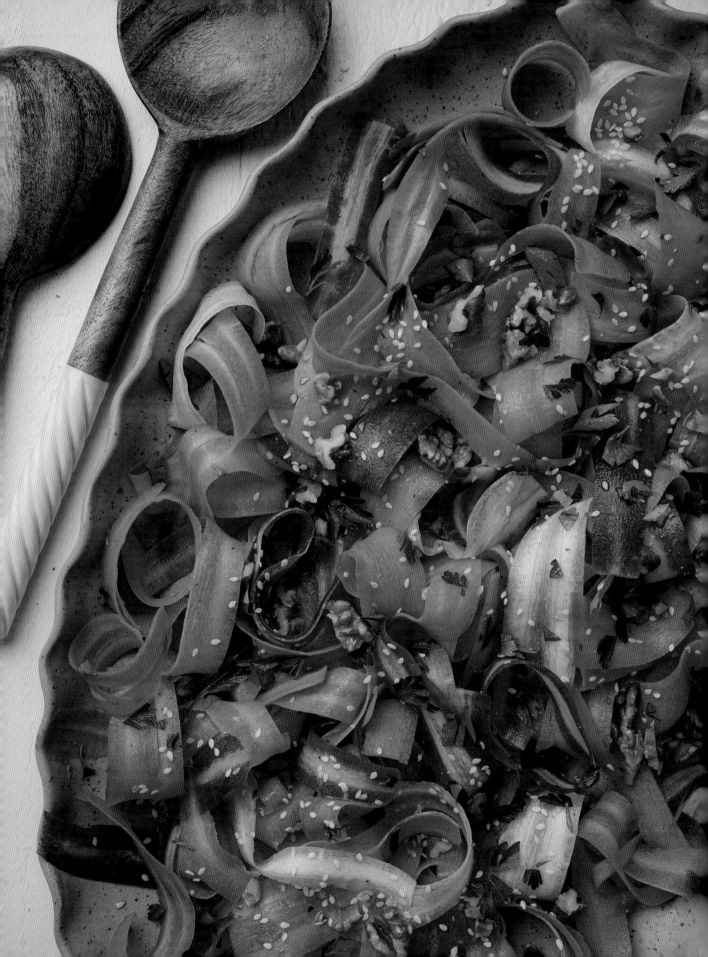

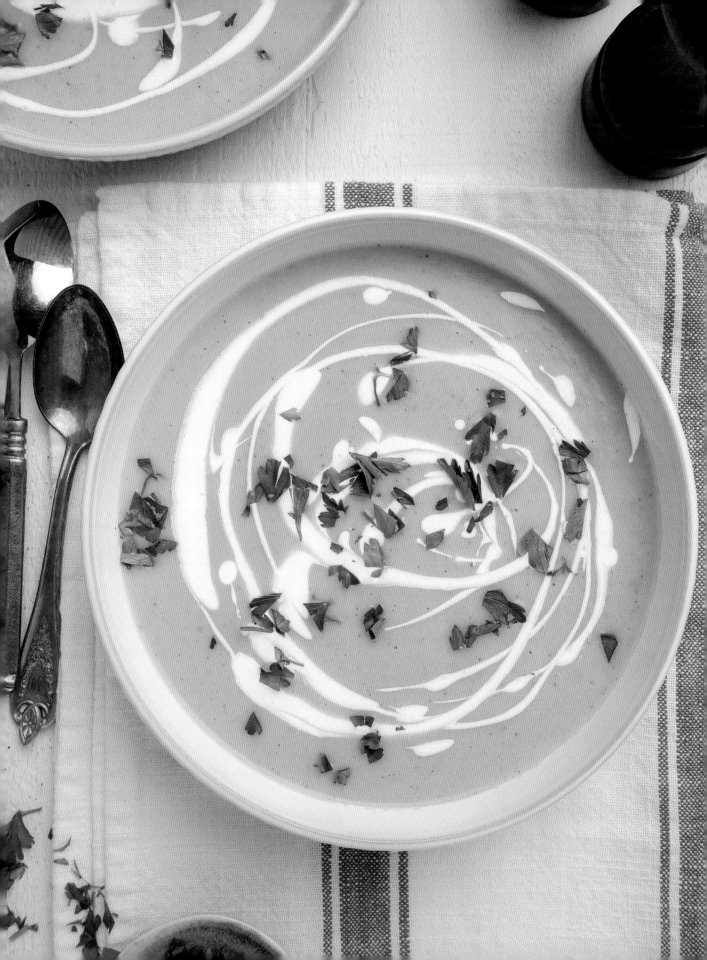

GINGER CARROT SOUP

Rachael: Pregnancy can come with its fair share of discomforts, so finding ways to provide comfort during the process is key. This may come in the form of a pregnancy pillow for when you can't sleep without support or, in our case here, a carrot ginger soup. In the colder months when you're feeling under the weather, there's nothing like a soup that warms the soul. I love the addition of ginger to this recipe, as it contains anti-inflammatory properties and can act as a digestive aid.

SERVINGS: 3–4	**PREP TIME:** 10 MINUTES	**TOTAL TIME:** 45 MINUTES

1 tablespoon olive oil or coconut oil

1 yellow onion, chopped

1 pound (450g) carrots, peeled and chopped

2 garlic cloves, minced

3 tablespoons minced fresh ginger

4 cups vegetable broth

1 (13.5-ounce/380g) can full-fat coconut milk

Salt and pepper, to taste

Fresh cilantro or parsley leaves, optional, for garnish

Plain coconut yogurt or Greek yogurt, optional, for serving

1. In a large pot, heat the olive oil over medium heat.
2. Add the onion and sauté until softened and translucent, about 5 minutes.
3. Add the carrots to the pot and stir to combine.
4. Stir in the garlic and ginger, and cook for an additional 1 to 2 minutes until fragrant.
5. Pour in the vegetable broth, ensuring that the carrots are fully submerged.
6. Bring the mixture to a boil, then reduce the heat to low and let it simmer, covered, for about 20 to 25 minutes or until the carrots are tender.
7. Once the carrots are cooked through, remove the pot from the heat.
8. Using an immersion blender, purée the soup until smooth and creamy. Alternatively, you can transfer the soup in batches to a blender and blend until smooth. Be cautious when blending hot liquids and don't overfill the blender.
9. Return the puréed soup to the pot if using a blender. Reduce the heat to low to keep the soup warm.
10. Stir in the coconut milk until well combined and season with salt and pepper to taste.
11. Serve the soup hot, garnished with fresh cilantro or parsley and a dollop of yogurt, if desired.

Note   *If the soup is too thick, you can add more vegetable broth or water to reach your desired consistency.*

CARROT FRIES
WITH DIPPING SAUCE

Rachael: Fries are a part of my love language, and I don't discriminate against any type of fries. Waffle fries, sweet potato fries, zucchini fries—I love them all. Today, we will be making carrot fries. I love knowing carrots are rich in vitamins too, so the baby will be getting some extra vitamin A, C, and B_6 in the process.

SERVINGS: 2–3	**PREP TIME:** 10 MINUTES	**TOTAL TIME:** 35 MINUTES

4 large carrots, peeled
2 tablespoons olive oil or avocado oil
1 teaspoon garlic powder
1 teaspoon paprika
½ teaspoon ground cumin
1 teaspoon flaky sea salt, plus more to taste
½ teaspoon black pepper, plus more to taste
Chopped fresh parsley or cilantro, for optional garnish

FOR THE DIPPING SAUCE
½ cup mayonnaise
Juice of a ½ lime (about 1 tablespoon)
2–3 dashes hot sauce
Sprinkle of diced chives

1 **Prepare the dipping sauce.** In a small cup or ramekin, mix together the mayonnaise, lime juice, and hot sauce. Cover and place in the fridge.

2 Preheat the oven to 425°F (220°C) and line a baking sheet with parchment paper or aluminum foil.

3 Cut the peeled carrots into a classic French-fry cut or *battonet*, which measures at least ¼ x ¼ x 2½ inches (6mm x 6mm x 6.25cm).

4 In a large mixing bowl, toss the carrot fries with olive oil until evenly coated.

5 Sprinkle the garlic powder, paprika, ground cumin, salt, and pepper over the carrot fries, and toss to coat evenly.

6 Arrange the seasoned carrot fries in a single layer on the prepared baking sheet, making sure they are not overcrowded. This will ensure even cooking and crispiness.

7 Place the baking sheet in the preheated oven and bake for 20 to 25 minutes or until the carrot fries are tender and golden brown, flipping halfway through the cooking time for even browning.

8 Once the carrot fries are cooked to your desired crispiness, remove them from the oven and check for seasoning and add additional salt and pepper to taste.

9 Transfer the carrot fries to a serving platter and garnish with chopped fresh parsley or cilantro, if desired.

10 Remove the dipping sauce from the fridge and sprinkle chives over the top. Serve alongside the fries.

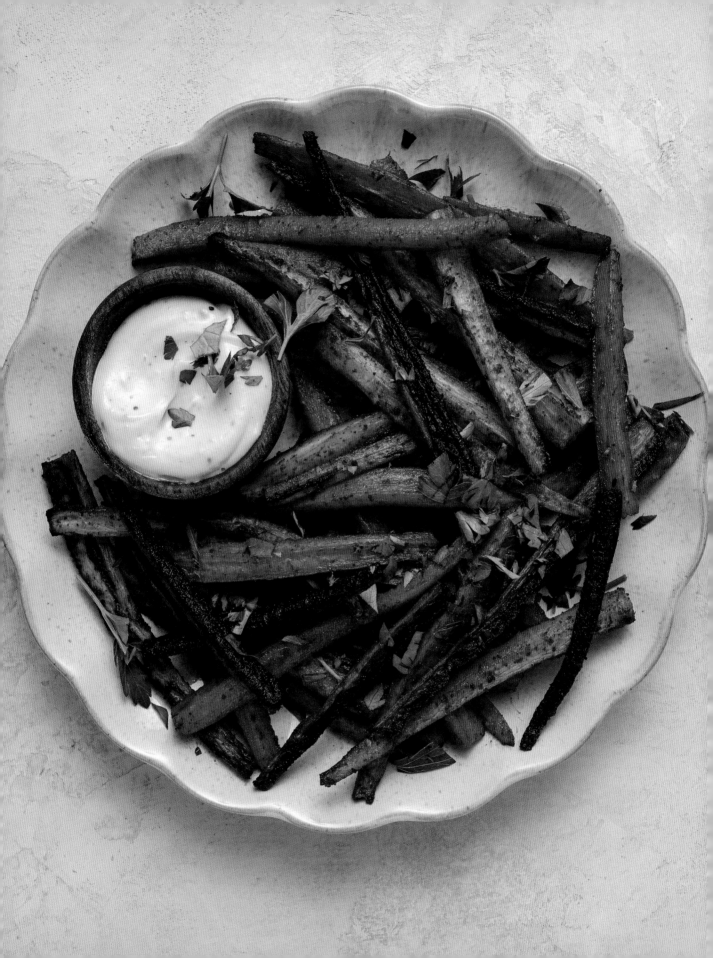

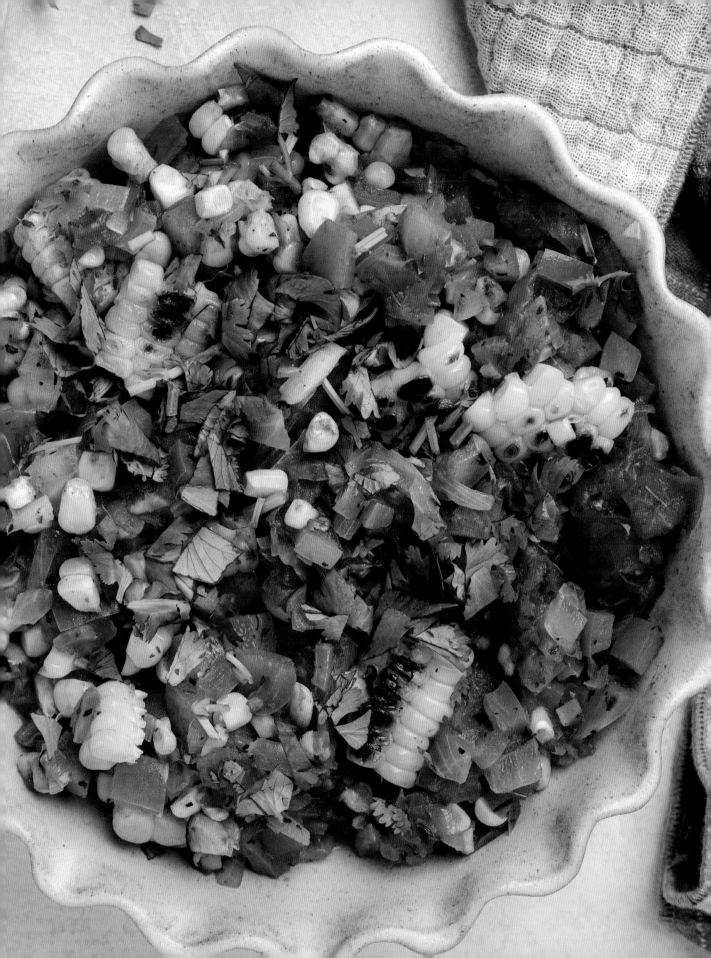

CHARRED-CORN MAQUE CHOUX

Rachael: Have you thought of baby names yet? If not, don't stress. It took us three days to name our daughter Sutton after she was born. (They wouldn't let us leave the hospital without a name, understandably.) There will be lots of names you find inspiration from and then find a way to make it uniquely your own. I love that creating recipes takes you through the same thought process. You take inspiration from dishes that already exist and make them your own. This recipe was Inspired by *maque choux*, a traditional dish from Louisiana, and we are taking inspiration from the flavors and turning it into a salad that also tastes delicious served over fish, chicken, or tacos.

SERVINGS: 4–6	**PREP TIME:** 10 MINUTES	**TOTAL TIME:** 40 MINUTES

4 ears fresh corn, husks and silk removed

2 tablespoons olive oil or avocado oil, divided

1 yellow onion, diced small

1 green bell pepper, diced small

2 garlic cloves, minced

2 heirloom tomatoes, diced small

1 teaspoon smoked paprika

½ teaspoon dried thyme

½ teaspoon dried oregano

Salt and pepper, to taste

Chopped fresh parsley or cilantro, optional, for garnish

1 Preheat a grill or grill pan over medium-high heat.

2 Brush the corn with 1 tablespoon of olive oil.

3 Place the corn on the grill and cook, turning occasionally, until charred on all sides, about 10 to 12 minutes. Remove from heat and let cool slightly.

4 Once cooled, use a knife to carefully slice the corn kernels off the cob. Set aside.

5 In a large skillet, heat 1 tablespoon of olive oil over medium heat. Add the onion and bell pepper, and sauté until softened, about 5 minutes.

6 Add the garlic to the skillet and cook for another 1 to 2 minutes, until fragrant.

7 Stir in the tomatoes, paprika, thyme, oregano, salt, and pepper. Cook for 5 minutes, until the tomatoes start to break down and release their juices.

8 Add the charred corn kernels to the skillet and stir to combine. Cook for an additional 5 minutes, until the corn is heated through and flavors are well combined.

9 Transfer the maque choux to a serving dish and garnish with chopped fresh parsley or cilantro, if desired.

10 Serve hot as a side dish or as a topping for grilled chicken, fish, or tacos.

CHARRED CORN & ONION CHOWDER

Rachael: How we feeling this week? There's the initial mob of people who will ask about how you are feeling after you announce and then it gets pretty quiet until you're at the tail-end of pregnancy. So if no one has asked how you are doing, let's pretend I'm with you and we are chatting over a bowl of this charred corn-and-onion chowder. If you are irritable and everything your partner says and does annoys you . . . I understand all too well. You may also be in such bliss that you just want to tell someone how truly happy you are without shoving it in their face. Whatever you need to get off your chest, I'm here to listen. My DMs are always open.

SERVINGS: 4–6	PREP TIME: 10 MINUTES	TOTAL TIME: 50 MINUTES

4 ears fresh corn, husks and silk removed

1 large yellow onion, sliced into thick rounds

2 tablespoons olive oil, divided

2 garlic cloves, minced

2 medium potatoes, peeled and diced

1 teaspoon smoked paprika

½ teaspoon dried thyme

Salt and pepper, to taste

4 cups vegetable broth

1 cup full-fat coconut milk

Chopped fresh parsley or chives, for garnish

1 Preheat a grill or grill pan to medium-high heat.

2 Brush the corn and onion rounds with olive oil, and place them directly on the hot grill or into the grill pan.

3 Grill the onion rounds for 5 to 6 minutes per side, until charred and softened. Grill the corn for 10 to 12 minutes, turning occasionally, until charred in spots and tender. Remove the onion and corn from the grill and let them cool slightly.

4 Using a knife, carefully cut the grilled corn kernels off the cobs and set aside. Chop the onions into 1-inch (2.5cm) pieces and set aside.

5 In a large pot, heat 1 tablespoon of olive oil over medium heat. Add the garlic and cook for 1 to 2 minutes until fragrant.

6 Add the chopped grilled onion, potatoes, paprika, thyme, salt, and pepper. Stir to combine and allow to cook for 3 to 4 minutes

7 Pour in the vegetable broth and coconut milk. Bring the mixture to a simmer. Simmer the chowder for about 15 to 20 minutes or until the potatoes are tender.

8 Add the reserved corn kernels to the pot and stir to combine. Cook for an 5 minutes more to heat through. Taste and adjust seasoning if needed with more salt and pepper.

9 For a creamier texture, you can blend a portion of the chowder using an immersion blender or regular blender. Be sure to leave some chunks for texture.

10 Ladle the chowder into bowls and garnish with chopped fresh parsley or chives before serving.

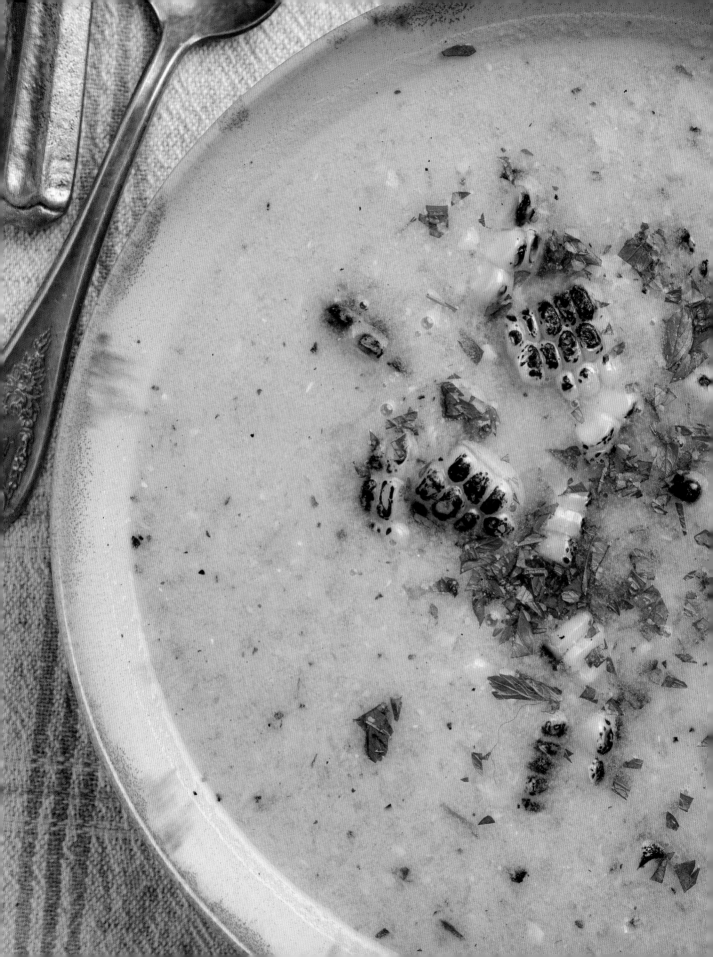

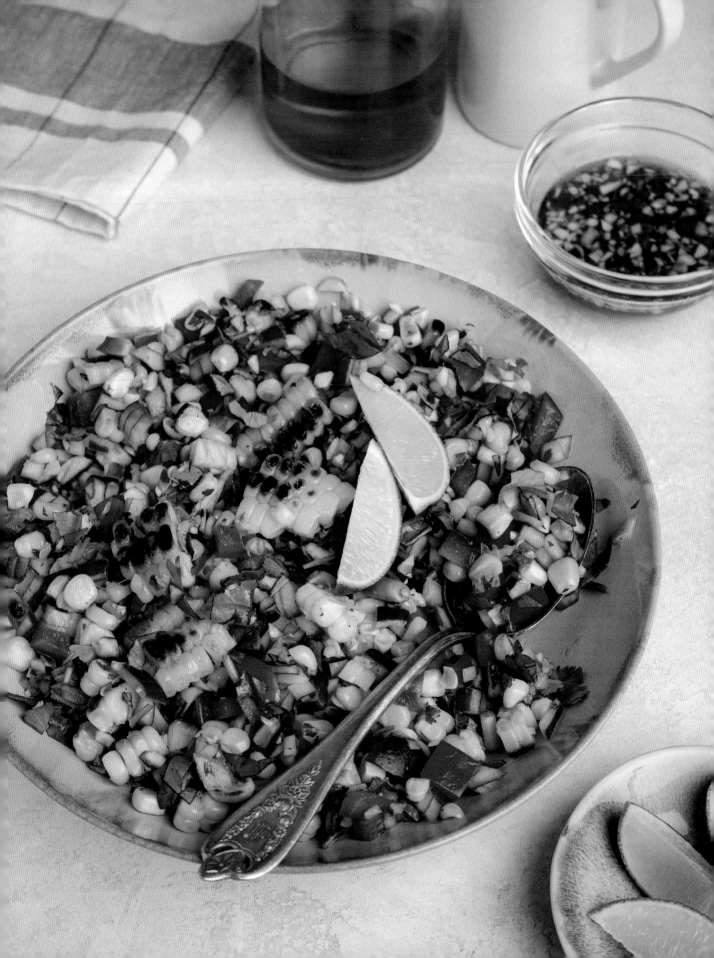

THAI STREET-CORN SALAD

Rachael: As you fade out of the honeymoon phase of pregnancy, aka the second trimester, and enter the third trimester, you may find yourself feeling extra tired and having trouble sleeping through the night. Thankfully, this salad is fairly quick and easy to put together, so you can still enjoy a yummy and nutritious meal without added stress and effort. Plus, this recipe gets bonus points from Tom because it stores nicely in the fridge for leftovers and makes a delicious midnight snack for those restless nights.

SERVINGS: 4	PREP TIME: 20 MINUTES	TOTAL TIME: 1 HOUR

4 ears corn, husks and silk removed
Olive oil, for brushing
1 red bell pepper, diced
¼ cup finely chopped red onion
¼ cup chopped fresh cilantro
¼ cup chopped fresh Thai basil
¼ cup chopped roasted peanuts, optional
Lime wedges, for serving

FOR THE DRESSING
Zest and juice of 1 lime
2 tablespoons fish sauce or tamari sauce
1 tablespoon honey or maple syrup
1 tablespoon olive oil
1 bird's-eye chili pepper or small chili pepper, finely chopped
1 garlic clove, minced
Salt and pepper, to taste

1 Preheat a grill or grill pan over medium-high heat.

2 Brush the corn on all sides with olive oil and place on the grill and cook, turning occasionally, until lightly charred on all sides, about 8 to 10 minutes. Remove from heat and let cool slightly.

3 Once cooled, use a knife to carefully slice the kernels off the cob. Place the kernels in a large mixing bowl.

4 Add the red bell pepper, red onion, cilantro, basil, and roasted peanuts (if using) to the bowl with the corn kernels.

5 **Make the dressing.** In a small bowl, whisk together all the dressing ingredients until well combined. Adjust seasoning with salt and pepper to taste.

6 Pour the dressing over the salad ingredients in the bowl.

7 Toss everything together until the salad is evenly coated with the dressing.

8 Cover the bowl and refrigerate for at least 30 minutes to allow the flavors to meld together.

9 Before serving, give the salad a final toss and adjust seasoning if necessary.

10 Serve the salad chilled with lime wedges on the side for squeezing over the top.

JICAMA CEVICHE
WITH JICAMA CHIPS

Rachael: During our babymoon, the chefs at the resort got wind of how Tom would make recipes that represented the baby's growth to celebrate our pregnancy, and they wanted to contribute to the series. To help make a special memory for us, they prepared an entire jicama-themed meal! From creating three courses around the vegetable to even making a special-themed mocktail, everything was jicama! This jicama ceviche was one of the courses they prepared for us. Not every recipe has a special story, but I love being able to share the ones that do.

SERVINGS: 6–8	PREP TIME: 15 MINUTES	TOTAL TIME: 45 MINUTES

2 cups peeled and diced jicama
1 cup quartered cherry tomatoes
½ red onion, finely diced
½ English cucumber, diced
1 avocado, diced
¼ cup chopped fresh cilantro
1 jalapeño, seeded and finely diced, optional
¼ cup fresh lime juice
Salt and pepper, to taste

FOR THE JICAMA CHIPS
1 large jicama, peeled and thinly sliced
Salt, to taste
2 tablespoons lime juice
2 tablespoons Tajin seasoning

1 **Prepare the jicama ceviche.** Place the diced jicama in a large mixing bowl. Add the cherry tomatoes, red onion, cucumber, avocado, cilantro, and jalapeño, if using.

2 Add the lime juice and gently toss all the ingredients together until well combined. Season with salt and pepper to taste

3 Cover the bowl with plastic wrap and refrigerate the jicama ceviche for at least 30 minutes to allow the flavors to meld together.

4 **Prepare the jicama chips while the ceviche chills.** Preheat the oven to 250°F (120°C) degrees and line a large baking sheet with parchment paper.

5 Peel the large jicama and thinly slice to ⅛-inch (3mm) thick using a mandoline slicer or a sharp knife.

6 In a medium bowl, add the jicama rounds with the salt, lime juice, and Tajin. Toss to coat evenly.

7 Arrange the jicama rounds in a single layer onto the prepared baking sheet.

8 Bake the jicama in the oven for 30 minutes or until the chips have crisped.

9 Remove from the oven and transfer to a wire rack to cool.

10 Serve the jicama ceviche in a bowl alongside with the jicama chips and enjoy!

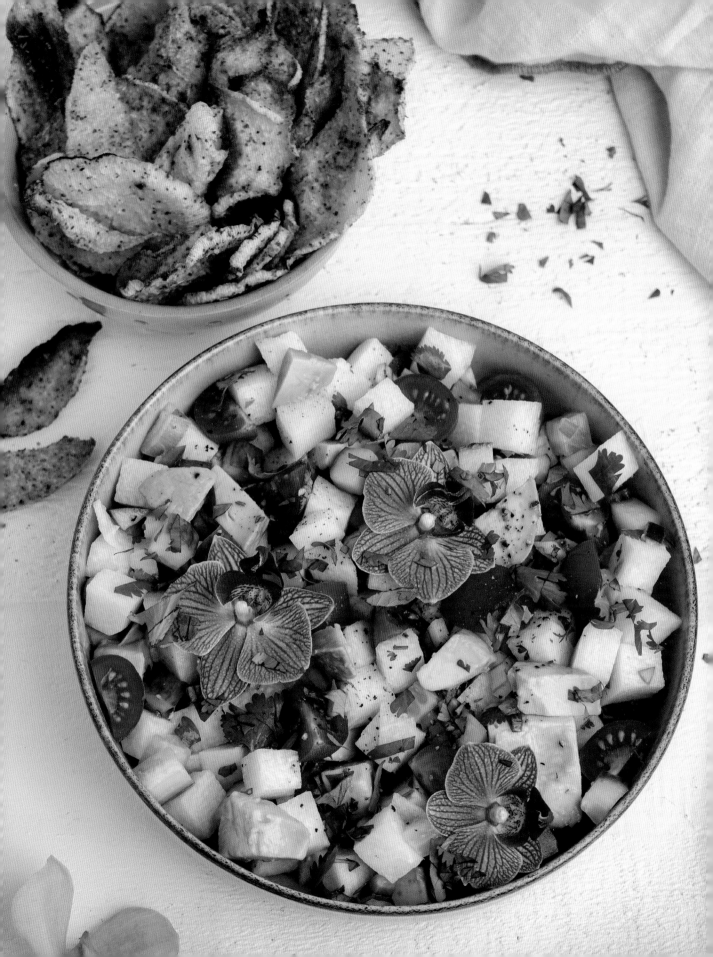

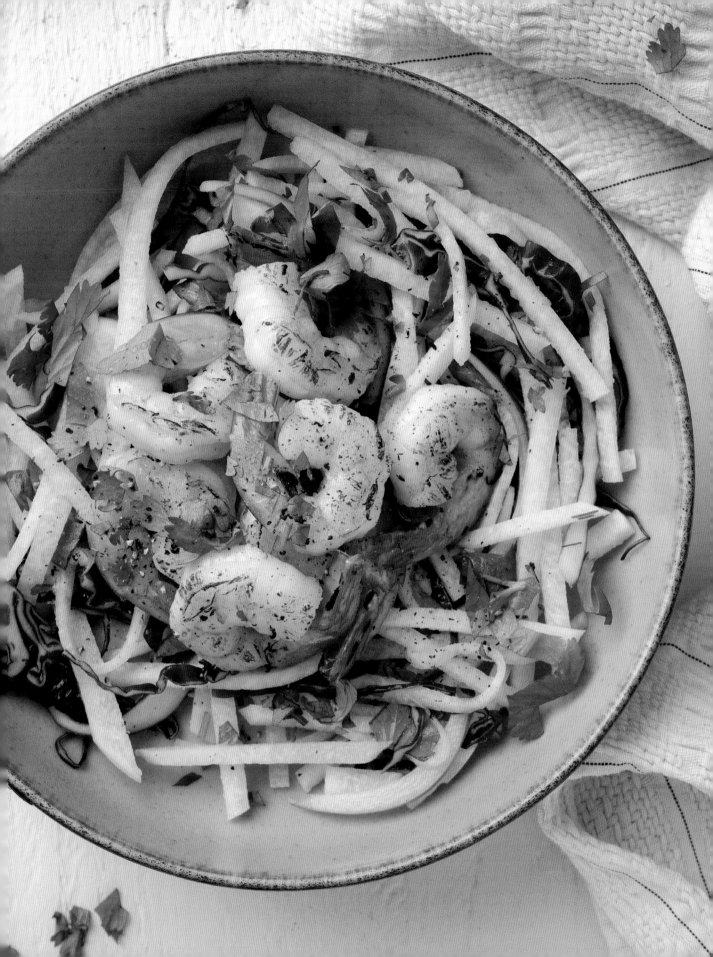

SAUTÉED SHRIMP

WITH JICAMA & CILANTRO SLAW

Rachael: There isn't only one way to parent, just like there isn't only one way to cook with an ingredient. One of my favorite things about this book is that every week we get to show you several ways to prepare the same fruit or vegetable. If you're in the same boat as me, I had never tried jicama until we started cooking for this series. It's a fun ingredient to incorporate into a slaw because it holds its texture, and a good crunch goes a long way. If you find yourself typically only having slaws with barbecue dishes, we can't wait to open your eyes and palette to the variety of ways to serve slaw starting with these sautéed shrimp.

SERVINGS: 4	**PREP TIME:** 40 MINUTES	**TOTAL TIME:** 50 MINUTES

2 tablespoons olive oil
2 garlic cloves, minced
2 tablespoons lime juice
Salt and pepper, to taste
1 pound (450g) large shrimp, peeled and deveined

FOR THE SLAW
2 tablespoons olive oil
2 tablespoons lime juice
1 tablespoon mayonnaise, or more to taste
1 tablespoon honey
2 tablespoons rice vinegar
1 large jicama, peeled and julienned
½ cup thinly sliced red cabbage
¼ cup chopped fresh cilantro, plus more for garnish
¼ cup thinly sliced red onion
Salt and pepper, to taste

1 To a medium bowl, add the olive oil, garlic, lime juice, salt, and pepper. Whisk to combine.

2 Add the shrimp to the bowl and toss to coat them evenly.

3 Cover the bowl and let the shrimp marinate in the fridge for 30 minutes.

4 **Prepare the slaw while the shrimp marinates.** In a large bowl, add the olive oil, lime juice, mayonnaise, honey and rice vinegar. Whisk to combine into a dressing.

5 Add in the jicama, red cabbage, cilantro, and red onion. Season with salt and pepper to taste. Toss to coat everything evenly and set aside to marinate while you cook the shrimp.

6 Heat a large skillet over medium-high heat. Add the marinated shrimp and cook for 2 to 3 minutes per side, or until the shrimp turn pink and are cooked through. Remove from the heat and set aside.

7 Arrange a portion of the jicama and cilantro slaw on a plate. Top the slaw with the sautéed shrimp.

8 Garnish with extra chopped cilantro. Serve and enjoy!

JICAMA FRIES
WITH CREAMY AVOCADO DIPPING SAUCE

Tom: Jicama fries with creamy avocado dipping sauce are a delicious twist on classic fries. They make a fantastic side dish, but let's be honest, if you eat an entire tray of fries for dinner, we won't tell. You can also rest easy knowing that jicama is rich in vitamin C and high in fiber, and the avocado dip adds a nice dose of healthy fats.

SERVINGS: 4	PREP TIME: 10 MINUTES	TOTAL TIME: 50 MINUTES

1 large jicama, peeled and cut into fries measuring ¼ x ¼ x 2½ inches (6mm x 6mm x 6.25cm)
2 tablespoons olive oil
1 teaspoon garlic powder
1 teaspoon paprika
½ teaspoon ground cumin
Salt and pepper, to taste

FOR THE CREAMY AVOCADO DIPPING SAUCE
1 ripe avocado
¼ cup plain coconut yogurt or Greek yogurt
1 tablespoon lime juice
1 garlic clove, minced
2 tablespoons chopped fresh cilantro
Salt and pepper, to taste

1 Bring a large pot of water to a boil.

2 Preheat the oven to 425°F (220°C), and line a large baking sheet with parchment paper.

3 Add the jicama fries to the pot of boiling water, and cook for about 10 minutes or until a paring knife inserted into the jicama gets little resistance.

4 Remove the jicama from the water and drain in a colander.

5 In a large bowl, add the drained jicama, olive oil, garlic powder, paprika, and cumin. Season with salt and pepper to taste and toss everything until evenly coated.

6 Arrange the seasoned jicama fries in a single layer on the prepared baking sheet.

7 Bake for 25 to 30 minutes, flipping halfway, until the fries are golden brown and crispy.

8 **Prepare the creamy avocado dipping sauce.** In a blender or food processor, combine all the dipping sauce ingredients. Blend until smooth and season with salt and pepper to taste.

9 Once the jicama fries are done baking, remove them from the oven and transfer them to a serving platter. Garnish with additional chopped fresh cilantro over the top, if desired.

10 Serve the jicama fries with the creamy avocado dipping sauce on the side and enjoy!

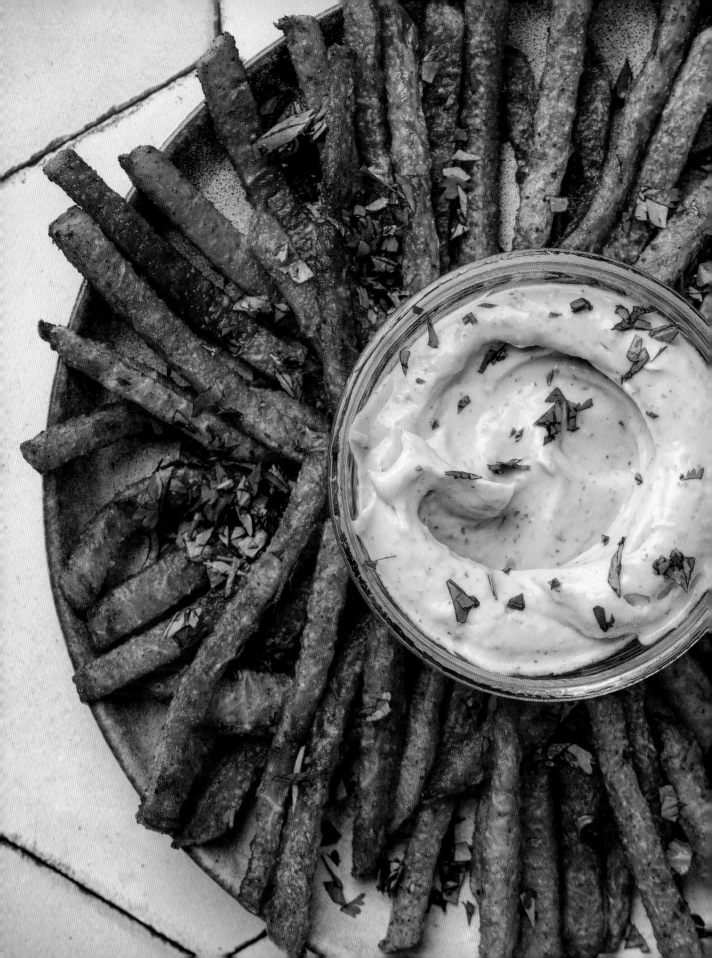

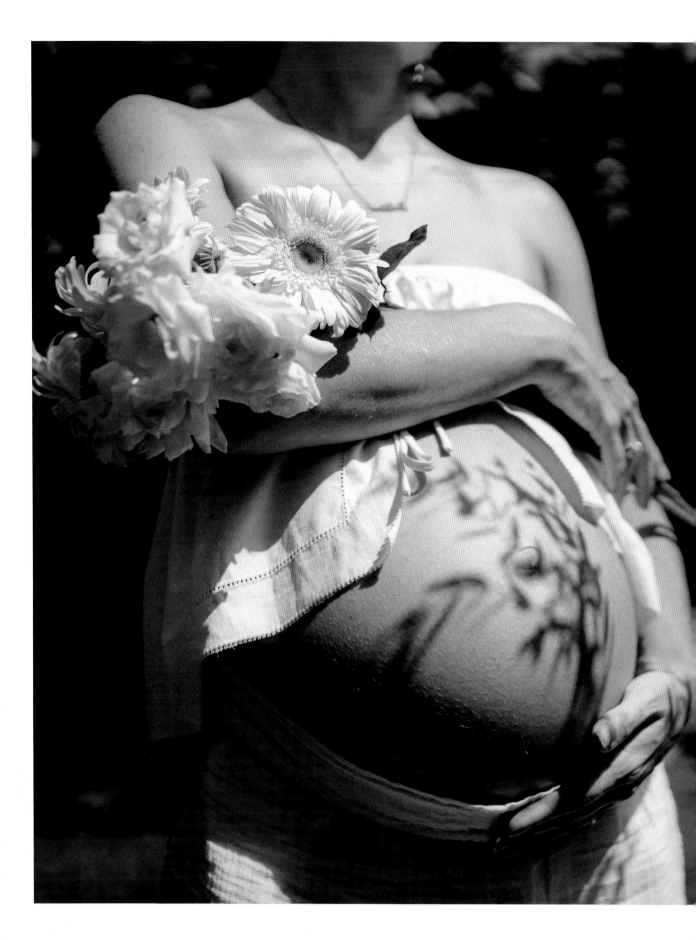

THIRD
TRIMESTER

*A*s you approach your due date, you are welcomed into the third trimester, a season of excitement and anticipation, as well as a season of readiness. Ready to have your body back, ready for your hormones to balance again, and overall ready to close a chapter on pregnancy and meet your baby. You have put in the hard work over the course of the last several months and the finish line is in sight. I want to take this moment to tell you how proud we are of you. Pregnancy is no easy feat for the mind, body, or soul. Be proud of your body and how it has grown, changed, and shaped itself to house this beautiful life, and most importantly, be proud of yourself, your strength, and how far you have come.

THIRD TRIMESTER MILESTONES

- Typically, the baby moves into a head-down position in preparation for birth. Or your baby may have their own plans and be stubborn, deciding to stay cozy in a different position— sometimes sideways or even feet-first.

- Your baby is now strong enough to grasp a finger, which means they'll also be strong enough to grasp your hair. Trust me, a ponytail will be your best friend.

- Inhaling, exhaling, and blinking are just a few of the new skills that your baby has been practicing.

- Your little one's hearing is now fully developed, so start chit chatting away because they may now be reacting to the sound of your voice.

SYMPTOMS YOU MAY EXPERIENCE

- Mask of pregnancy (melasma) (If you get the melasma mustache, consider it 24/7 lip liner.)
- Stretch marks (aka angel scratches)
- Colostrum (leaky breasts)
- Pregnancy rage (If you're feeling a little angry and irritable, like the "little things" are more difficult to handle . . . I was there with you.)
- Fast-growing hair
- Insomnia (Which makes for great late-night shopping.)
- Nesting instinct
- Mucus plug falls out (This has never happened to me, so I have no advice, but good luck!)

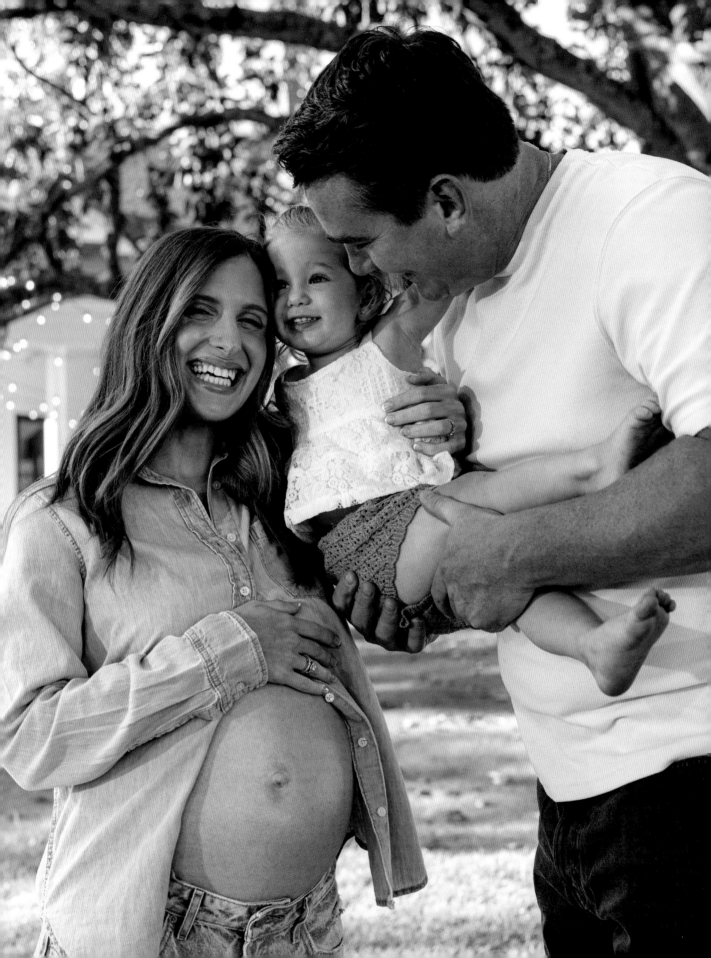

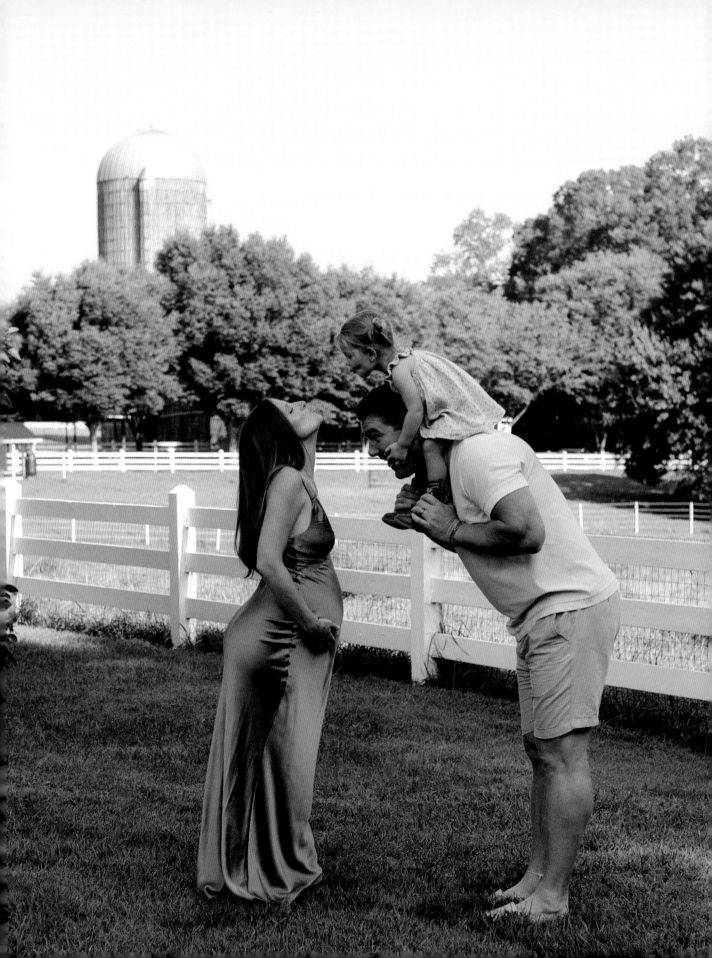

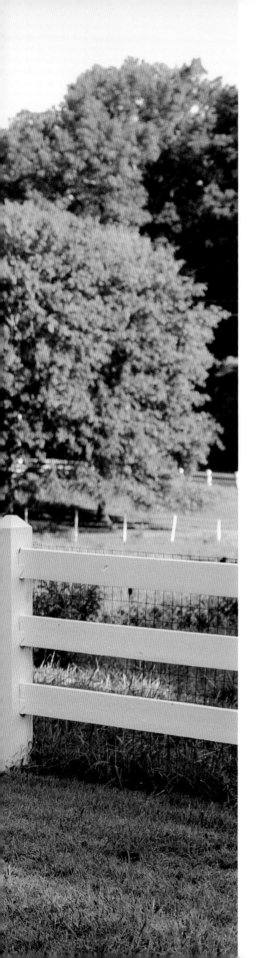

WAYS TO PREPARE FOR THIS SEASON

You might be starting to hear about all the "just wait until" moments. You probably have experienced this already: friends, family, and random strangers fall into two groups of "just wait until," followed by either something amazing to look forward to or a dramatization of impending doom. For example, "You guys better get all your sleep in; just wait, that won't be happening anymore." Let us remind you of all the amazing things that are to come. Just wait until you meet your baby for the first time, see their smile, listen to their laugh. Just wait until you watch your partner hold them. Just wait until you match as a family and introduce them to their siblings. This is not a season to fear, but rather embrace all the goodness that is to come.

While you are patiently waiting for those special first moments with your baby, take the time to cherish the last remaining weeks of your pregnancy. Document the end of your journey with maternity photos. If you're not in nesting mode already, start to prepare your home for the baby's arrival. Pack your hospital bag, build a postpartum cart . . . do whatever the word "comfort" means for you. If you have other children, make intentional time as a family because, as you know, these moments are fleeting.

ROASTED GRAPE & RED ONION PORK

Tom: If you have never roasted grapes before, I can promise you one thing—you will try and find ways to incorporate them into more meals. This dish is very simple and inexpensive but remains elegant. Perfect for celebrating a special occasion, such as being in week 27, which means the baby can hear your voice now.

SERVINGS: 2–4	**PREP TIME:** 15 MINUTES	**TOTAL TIME:** 40 MINUTES

1 pound (450g) pork tenderloin, trimmed and silverskin removed

Salt and pepper, to taste

2 cups red seedless grapes

1 large red onion, sliced

2 tablespoons coconut oil, melted

1 tablespoon fresh thyme, plus more for garnish

1 Preheat the oven to 400°F (200°C).

2 Pat the pork tenderloin dry with paper towels and season with salt and pepper on all sides.

3 On a large sheet pan, toss the grapes and red onion with the melted coconut oil, thyme, and additional salt and pepper until well coated.

4 Place the seasoned pork tenderloin on the pan along with the grape and onion mixture. Roll the pork tenderloin on the sheet to pick up some of the oil from the pan

5 Roast in the preheated oven for 20 to 25 minutes or until the pork reaches an internal temperature of 145°F (63°C) and the grapes and onions are caramelized and some of the grapes have burst open.

6 Remove the roasting pan from the oven and let the pork rest for 5 to 10 minutes before slicing.

7 Slice the pork into medallions and serve with the roasted grapes and red onions, along with the juices.

8 Garnish with additional fresh thyme, if desired, for an extra pop of flavor.

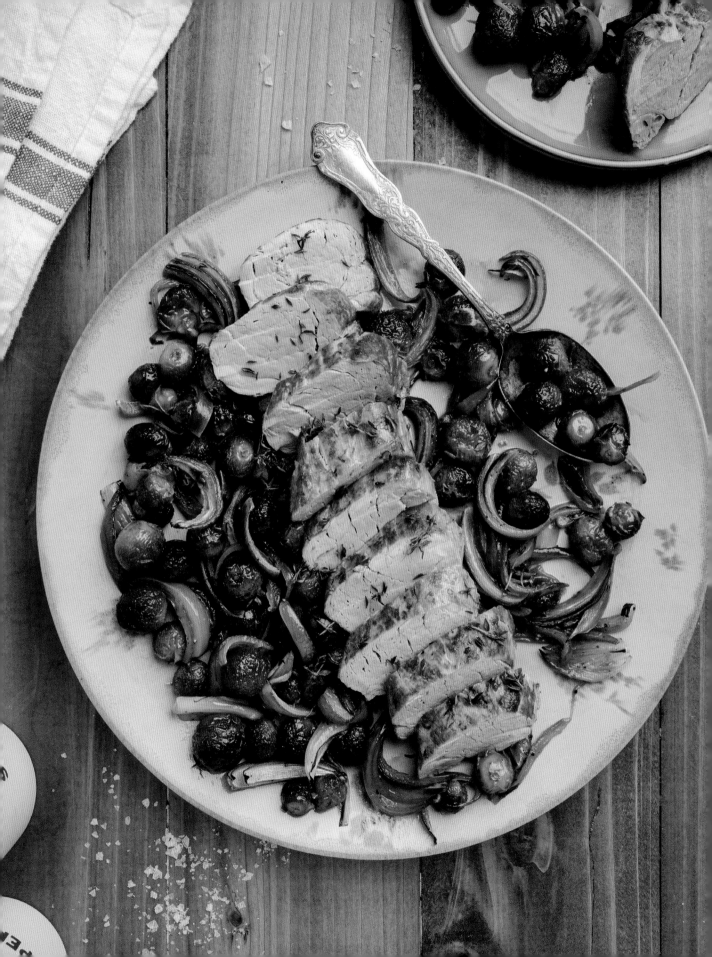

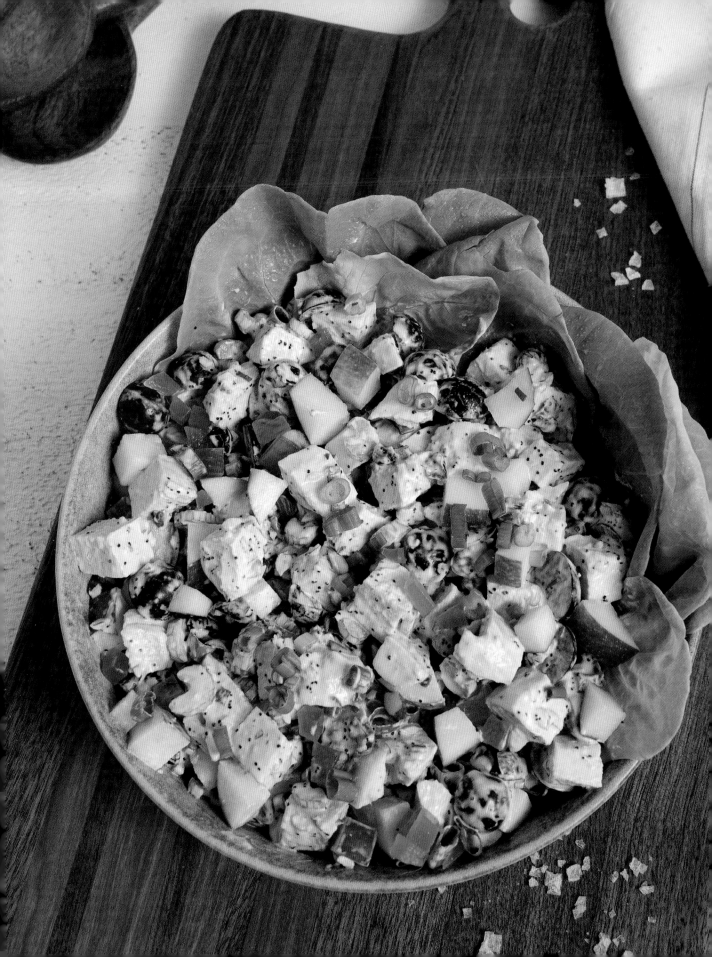

— week 27 —

SONOMA CHICKEN SALAD

Rachael: I will be very honest when I say we don't keep grapes in our home unless a recipe calls for it. Our first born, Odin, can't eat grapes because they could send him into kidney failure, because they are very toxic to dogs. Yes, you read that right. Our first born will always be our fur baby, and his needs come before my own. I also dealt with a lot of postpartum anxiety and struggled with the fear of my second born choking on grapes. With all that said, some of my favorite lunches, like this Sonoma chicken salad, include grapes. I used to pack this in my lunch box as a flight attendant, and it will forever have some of my favorite flavors and crunch all packed into one.

SERVINGS: 4	PREP TIME: 20 MINUTES	TOTAL TIME: 30 MINUTES

2 cups cooked chicken breast, shredded or diced
1 cup halved red seedless grapes
1 tablespoon poppy seeds
½ cup chopped celery
¼ cup chopped pecans or almonds
¼ cup chopped green onions
¼ cup dried cranberries, optional

FOR THE DRESSING
½ cup plain Greek yogurt
2 tablespoons mayonnaise
1 tablespoon Dijon mustard
1 tablespoon honey or maple syrup
1 tablespoon apple cider vinegar
½ teaspoon garlic powder
Salt and pepper, to taste

SERVING OPTIONS
Lettuce leaves or mixed greens
Chopped nuts
Green onions
Diced apples
Avocado
Dried apricots

1 **Prepare the salad.** In a large bowl, add the chicken, grapes, poppy seeds, celery, nuts, green onions, and cranberries (if using). Mix well to combine.

2 **Make the dressing.** In a small bowl, whisk together all the dressing ingredients until smooth and creamy.

3 Pour the dressing over the chicken salad mixture. Gently toss until all ingredients are evenly coated with the dressing. Check for seasoning and add additional salt and pepper to taste.

4 Cover the bowl and refrigerate for at least 30 minutes to allow the flavors to meld.

5 **To serve,** line a serving platter or individual plates with lettuce leaves or mixed greens. Spoon the chilled chicken salad onto the lettuce leaves or greens.

6 Garnish with additional chopped nuts or green onions, if desired.

7 Feel free to customize the salad with additional ingredients such as diced apples, avocado, or dried apricots, based on your preference.

— week 27 —

GRAPE HARVEST CRISP

Tom: You will be hearing a lot about oats when it comes to pregnancy, specifically during postpartum if you choose to breastfeed. Oats are generally recommended during pregnancy and postpartum to support overall health, energy levels, and enhance milk production. With that said, let's have some oats in a delicious dessert that has a short prep time and straightforward baking instructions.

SERVINGS: 3–5	**PREP TIME:** 10 MINUTES	**TOTAL TIME:** 45 MINUTES

2 cups halved fresh seedless grapes, any color
2 tablespoons honey or maple syrup
1 tablespoon cornstarch or arrowroot powder
1 tablespoon lemon juice
1 teaspoon ground cinnamon
1 teaspoon vanilla extract

FOR THE TOPPING
1 cup gluten-free rolled oats
½ cup almond flour
¼ cup chopped almonds or pecans chopped
¼ cup coconut sugar or brown sugar
¼ cup coconut oil, melted, plus more for greasing the pan
1 teaspoon ground cinnamon
Pinch of salt

SERVING OPTIONS
Vanilla or vanilla bean dairy-free ice cream or your preferred ice cream
Seedless grape halves

1 Preheat the oven to 350°F (180°C). Lightly grease an 8x8-inch (20x20cm) baking dish with coconut oil or cooking spray.

2 In a medium bowl, combine the grapes, honey, cornstarch, lemon juice, cinnamon, and vanilla extract and then toss until the grapes are evenly coated.

3 **Prepare the topping.** In another medium bowl, combine the topping ingredients and mix until well combined and crumbly.

4 Spread the grape filling evenly into the prepared baking dish.

5 Sprinkle the crisp topping over the grape filling, covering it completely.

6 Bake uncovered for 30 to 35 minutes or until the filling is bubbly and the topping is golden brown.

7 Remove the baking dish from the oven and let it cool for a few minutes before serving.

8 Serve warm, topped with your preferred ice cream. Garnish with additional fresh grapes if desired.

Note *Feel free to customize this recipe by substituting other fruits for the filling, such as strawberries or raspberries, based on your preference.*

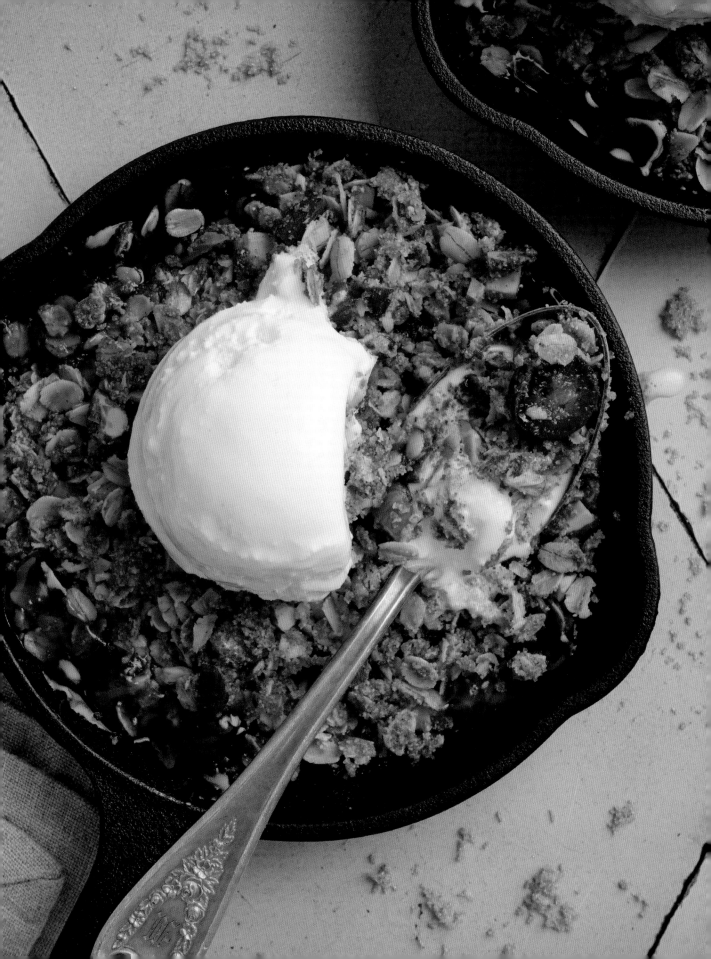

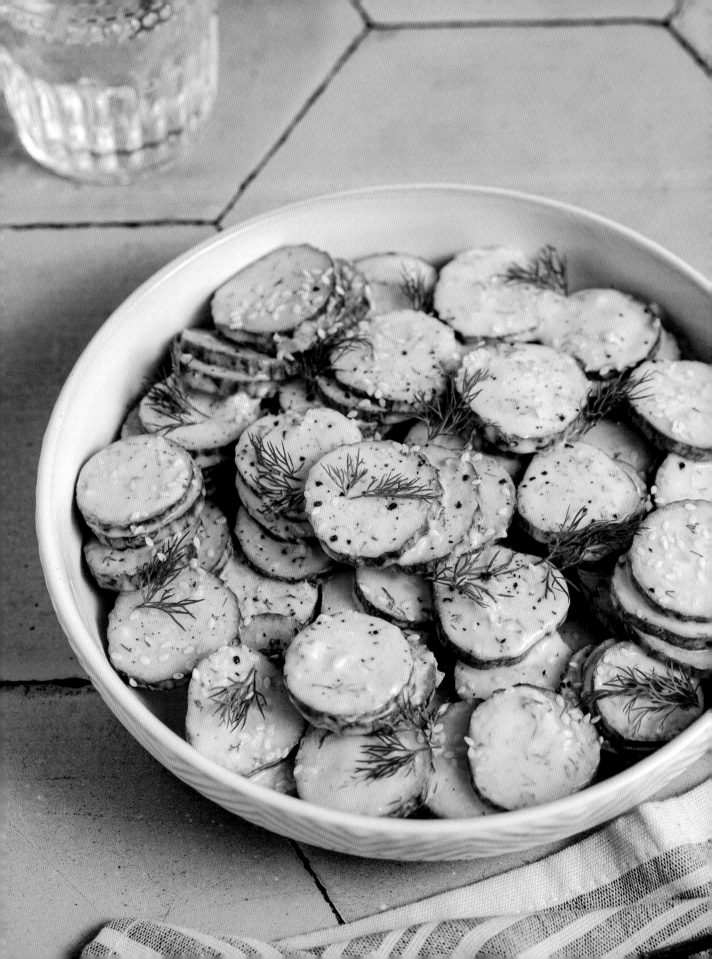

CUCUMBER TAHINI SALAD

Tom: This cucumber tahini salad is the perfect combination of simplicity and nutrition. Cucumbers, known for aiding digestion and hydration, form the crisp and refreshing base of this salad. The tahini dressing, rich in calcium, iron, and magnesium, provides essential minerals vital for both you and baby. With a quick prep time, this dish makes the perfect snack or addition as a side to a larger meal.

SERVINGS: 4–6	**PREP TIME:** 10 MINUTES	**TOTAL TIME:** 40 MINUTES

¼ cup tahini
2 tablespoons lemon juice
1 tablespoon olive oil
1 garlic clove, minced
1 tablespoon chopped fresh dill
Salt and pepper, to taste
2 large English cucumbers, sliced into rounds
Sesame seeds, optional
Chopped fresh parsley, optional

1 In a small bowl, whisk together the tahini, lemon juice, olive oil, garlic, and fresh dill until smooth and well combined. Season with salt and pepper to taste. You can adjust the consistency of this dressing by adding a little water if needed.

2 Place the sliced cucumbers in a large mixing bowl.

3 Pour the tahini dressing over the cucumbers and toss until they are evenly coated.

4 Cover the bowl and refrigerate the cucumber salad for at least 30 minutes to allow the flavors to meld and the cucumbers to marinate.

5 Once chilled, transfer the cucumber tahini salad to a serving dish.

6 If desired, garnish with sesame seeds and chopped fresh parsley.

CUCUMBER SALSA VERDE
WITH SHRIMP

Rachael: There is a huge chance that you don't even read this description because the sight of shrimp makes you queasy. This is why each week has several recipes, because we have a lot of cravings and aversions we are trying to satisfy. For those of you still with me because shrimp is a food you enjoy, we are pairing it this week with a cucumber salsa verde. Most of you are probably used to dipping your shrimp into cocktail sauce, so this idea is similar, except we are making a salsa . . . so I highly recommend including a handful of chips to scoop up the remaining dip with!

SERVINGS: 4	PREP TIME: 15 MINUTES	TOTAL TIME: 20 MINUTES

2 large cucumbers, chopped

4 tomatillos, husks removed and chopped

½ cup chopped fresh cilantro

½ white onion, chopped

1 jalapeño, ribs and seeds removed, roughly chopped

1 garlic clove

Juice of 1 lime

1 tablespoon olive oil

Salt and pepper, to taste

FOR THE SHRIMP

1 pound (450g) large shrimp, peeled and deveined

1 tablespoon olive oil

1 teaspoon ground cumin

1 teaspoon chili powder

Salt and pepper, to taste

SERVING OPTIONS

Fresh cilantro leaves

Lime wedges

1 In a blender, combine the cucumbers, tomatillos, cilantro, onion, jalapeño, garlic, lime juice, and olive oil. Blend until smooth.

2 Taste the salsa and season with salt and pepper to taste.

3 Once well seasoned, refrigerate the salsa while you prepare the shrimp.

4 **Prepare the shrimp.** In a separate bowl, toss the peeled and deveined shrimp with olive oil, ground cumin, chili powder, salt, and pepper until evenly coated.

5 Heat a large skillet over medium-high heat.

6 Add the seasoned shrimp to the skillet in a single layer.

7 Cook the shrimp for 2 to 3 minutes on each side, until pink and opaque.

8 Remove the skillet from the heat and set aside.

9 To serve, spoon the chilled cucumber salsa verde onto plates and top with the cooked shrimp.

10 Garnish the dish with additional cilantro leaves and lime wedges, if desired.

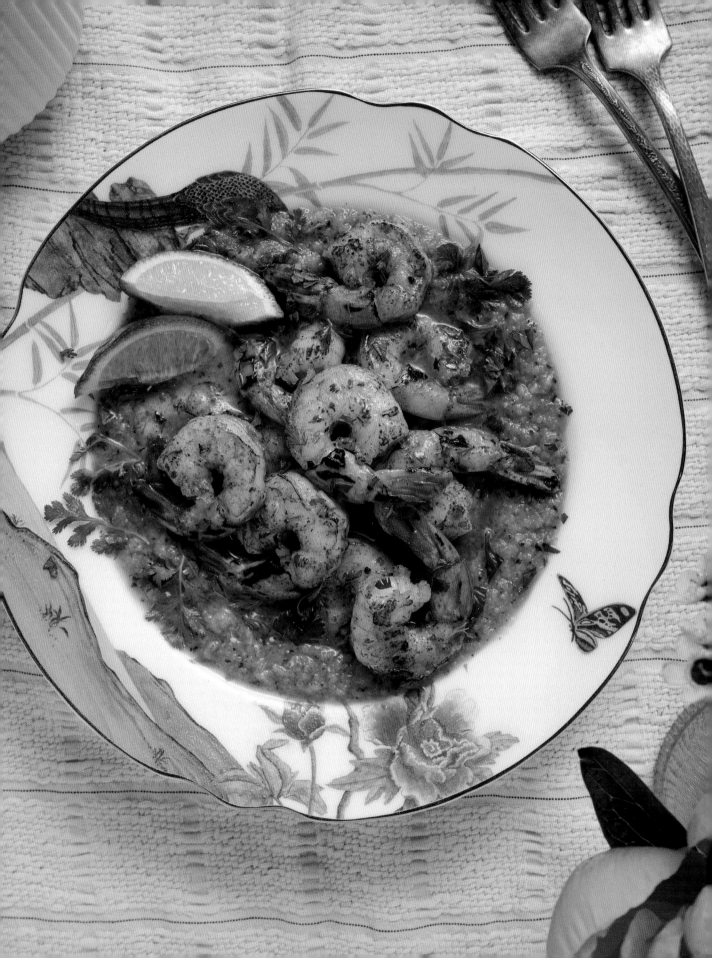

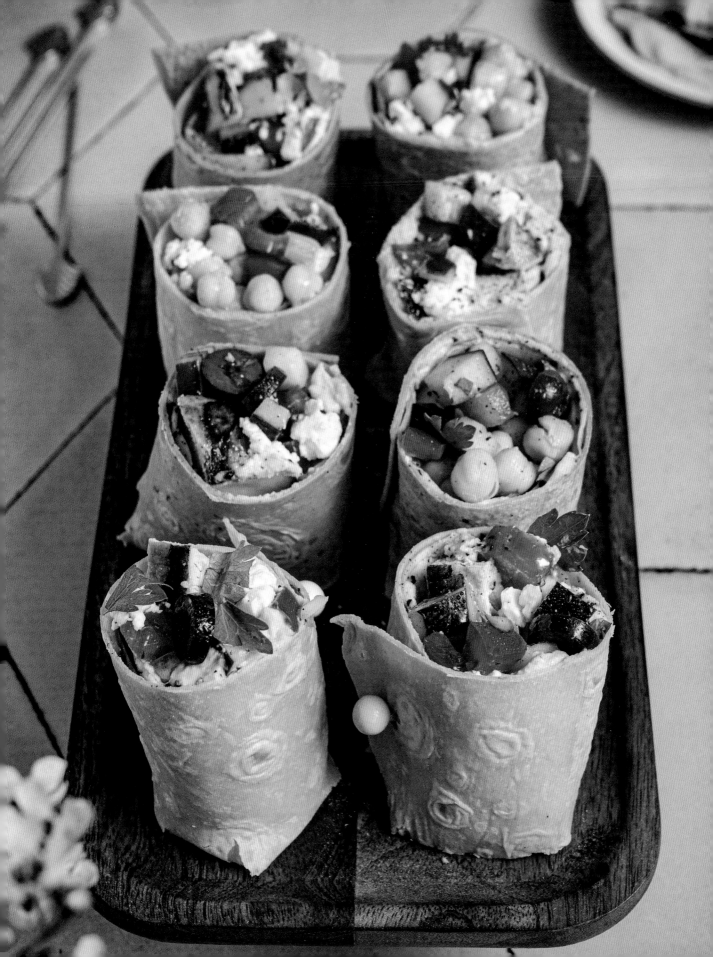

— week 28 —

MEDITERRANEAN CUCUMBER WRAP

Tom: You are about two-thirds of the way through your pregnancy and soon you are going to have to put those swaddle skills to the ultimate test! Because practice makes perfect, you can practice your swaddling skills by wrapping up a delicious variety of ingredients and enjoying this Mediterranean cucumber wrap.

SERVINGS: 2	PREP TIME: 15 MINUTES	TOTAL TIME: 15 MINUTES

2 large collard green leaves or gluten-free tortillas
¼ cup diced tomato
¼ cup diced English cucumber, plus 1 large English cucumber, peeled and thinly sliced lengthwise, used separately
¼ cup diced red bell pepper
¼ cup diced red onion
2 tablespoons chopped Kalamata olives
1 tablespoon chopped fresh parsley
1 tablespoon lemon juice
½ tablespoon olive oil
Pinch of salt and pepper or to taste
½ cup hummus

SERVING OPTIONS
¼ cup crumbled feta cheese
Grilled chicken
Chickpeas
Tofu strips

1 If using collard green leaves, wash and dry them thoroughly. Trim the tough stem at the base of each leaf. You can also lightly steam or blanch the collard green leaves to make them more pliable.

2 In a mixing bowl, combine ¼ cup diced English cucumber, bell pepper, red onion, kalamata olives, chopped parsley, lemon juice, olive oil and a pinch of salt and pepper. Toss to combine.

3 Lay out the collard green leaves on a flat surface.

4 Spread a generous layer of hummus evenly over each collard green leaf, leaving a border around the edges.

5 Place a layer of thinly sliced English cucumber strips on top of the hummus.

6 Spoon the prepared vegetable mixture evenly over the cucumber.

7 If desired, add crumbled feta, grilled chicken, chickpeas, or tofu strips on top of the filling for added protein.

8 Roll up the collard green leaves tightly around the filling, tucking in the sides as you go, and securing the wraps with toothpicks if needed.

9 Slice each wrap in half, serve, and enjoy!

— week 28 —

CUCUMBER MARGARITA MOCKTAIL

Rachael: Pregnancy is a never-ending quest for me to find and create the best mocktail. To be honest though, I always find myself going back to some variation of a margarita. So if you liked the spicy margarita we made when the baby was the size of a lime, honeyyyyy, we're back! This margarita in particular gives off refreshing spa-energy vibes. I like to think it's the type of drink they offer you to sip while you're relaxing in a meditation room before getting a massage. Cheers!

SERVINGS: 2	PREP TIME: 15 MINUTES	TOTAL TIME: 15 MINUTES

1 large cucumber, peeled and chopped
¼ cup fresh lime juice
2 tablespoons honey or agave syrup
¼ cup fresh mint leaves, plus extra for garnish

FOR SERVING
Lime wedges
Tajín seasoning or salt, optional
Ice cubes
Sparkling water or soda water, to top each glass
Fresh mint leaves

1 In a blender, combine the cucumber, lime juice, honey, and mint leaves.

2 Blend until smooth and well combined.

3 Strain the mixture through a fine-mesh sieve or cheesecloth to remove any pulp. You should have about 1 cup of cucumber juice.

4 **Serve your mocktail.** If desired, rim the edges of serving glasses with salt. To do this, rub a lime wedge around the rim of each glass, then dip the rim into a shallow dish of salt.

5 Fill the glasses with ice cubes. Divide the cucumber juice evenly among the prepared glasses.

6 Top each glass with sparkling water or soda water, stirring gently to combine.

7 Garnish each glass with a sprig of fresh mint and a lime wedge.

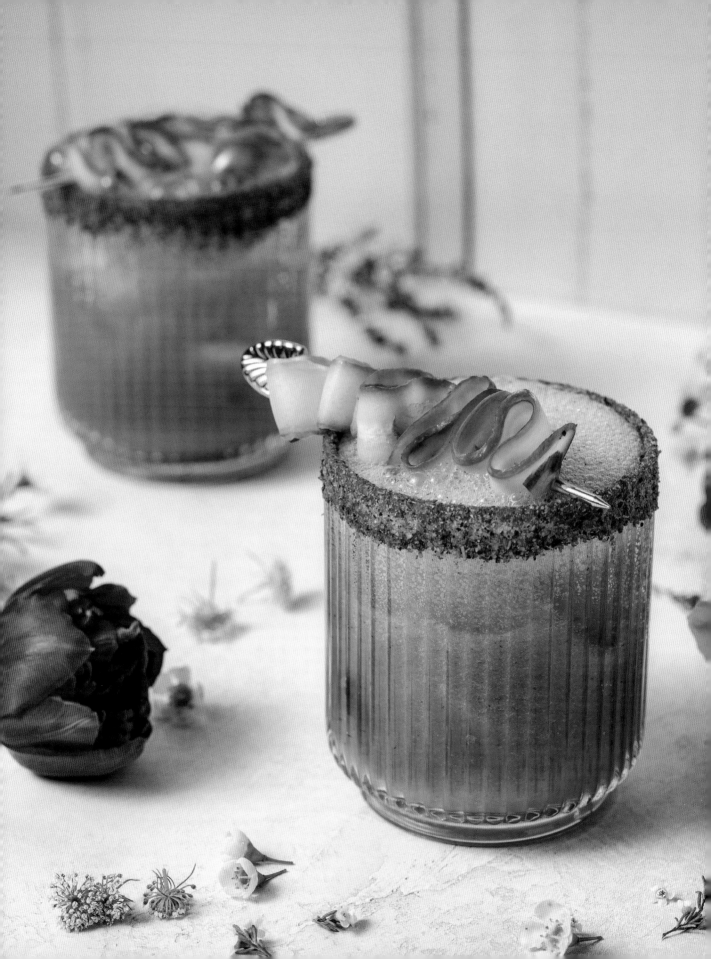

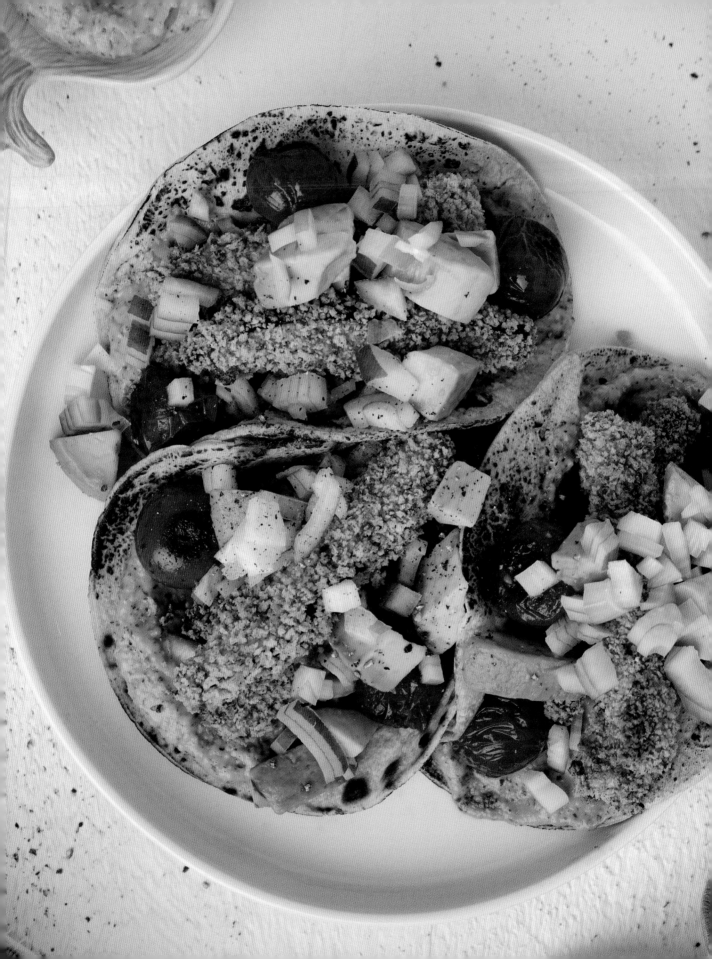

CRISPY EGGPLANT TACOS

Rachael: The first time we made eggplant tacos was at the very beginning of our fertility journey. I was skeptical to say the least. At this point the most "out of the box" taco creation Tom had made were his cauliflower tacos, but eggplant was in season and I was in a taco mood. They were unexpectedly delicious and have become a fan favorite amongst our vegetarian friends.

SERVINGS: 4	**PREP TIME:** 25 MINUTES	**TOTAL TIME:** 55 MINUTES

1 large eggplant
½ cup fine almond flour
2 large eggs whisked
1 cup gluten-free panko
2 teaspoons taco seasoning
Avocado oil or oil spray
1 cup halved cherry tomatoes
8 corn tortillas
1 avocado, diced
1 red onion, finely diced or pickled

FOR THE SAUCE
6 garlic cloves
1 large serrano pepper or jalapeño; ribs,
   seeds, and stems removed
1 cup fresh cilantro
¾ cup fresh parsley
½ ripe avocado
½ teaspoon salt
Juice of 1 lime
1 tablespoon agave syrup or honey
2–3 tablespoons avocado oil

1 **Prepare the sauce.** Add all the sauce ingredients to a food processor and process until nearly smooth. You may need to stop and use a spatula to scrape down any mixture collecting on the sides. Add more avocado oil or agave syrup as needed to thin the sauce. Refrigerate sauce until ready to use.

2 **Make the eggplant filling.** Preheat the oven to 425°F (220°C). Cut the eggplant into a classic French-fry cut or batonnet, which measures at least ¼ x ¼ x 2½ inches (6mm x 6mm x 6.25cm).

3 Prepare three small bowls. Fill one with the fine almond flour, one with the whisked eggs, and one with the panko and taco seasoning mixed together. Prepare a baking sheet with parchment paper. Spray or drizzle with avocado oil as needed.

4 Working in batches with a few pieces at a time, coat the eggplant with almond flour, shaking off any excess. Next dip into the whisked eggs. Then fully coat the eggplant pieces with the panko mixture. Place the battered eggplant on the prepared baking sheet. Repeat with the remaining eggplant.

5 Place the halved tomatoes evenly spaced on the same baking sheet next to the eggplant.

6 Bake the eggplant and tomatoes for 20 to 25 minutes, then increase the oven heat to 450°F (230°C) and bake for 5 more minutes or until the panko turns brown and crispy. You may need to remove the tomatoes early if they have sufficiently blistered.

7 **Build the tacos.** Warm the tortillas in the microwave, spread a spoonful of sauce on each, then add baked eggplant, diced avocado, diced onion, blistered tomatoes, and, if desired, top with more sauce.

— week 29 —

EGGPLANT DIP

Rachael: The only exposure I had to Mediterranean cuisine while growing up was the gyros served at a hamburger joint that I would ride my bike to during the summer. In the beginning of our marriage, Tom and I lived in downtown Chicago, where we were introduced to a wide variety of new foods from many different cultures. Because it took me nearly 25 years to try Mediterranean food, we are going to expand this child's palette early (as in "still in the womb") with some Mediterranean flavors. Hummus is the traditional dip we all know and love, so let us turn you on to eggplant dip (aka *baba ganoush*). It's amazing served with pita and vegetables as an appetizer or as a side dip to a fun bowl!

SERVINGS: 2–3	PREP TIME: 10 MINUTES	TOTAL TIME: 1 HOUR 30 MINUTES

1 large eggplant
2 tablespoons olive oil
2 garlic cloves, minced
1 tablespoon tahini
2 tablespoons lemon juice
1 teaspoon ground cumin
1 teaspoon smoked paprika
Salt and pepper, to taste

SERVING OPTIONS
Chopped fresh parsley
Smoked paprika
Extra-virgin olive oil
Gluten-free crackers
Gluten-free bread
Sliced fresh vegetables

Note *Feel free to adjust the seasonings and add additional herbs or spices according to your taste preferences. You can also experiment with different toppings or mix-ins, such as roasted red peppers or sun-dried tomatoes, to customize the flavor of the dip.*

1 Preheat the oven to 400°F (200°C).

2 Pierce the eggplant several times with a fork to allow steam to escape during roasting.

3 Place the whole eggplant on a baking sheet lined with parchment paper.

4 Roast for 40 to 45 minutes or until the eggplant is completely soft and collapsed. The skin should be charred and easily peel away. Once the eggplant is roasted, remove it from the oven and let it cool slightly.

5 Once cool enough to handle, cut the eggplant in half lengthwise and scoop out the flesh into a bowl, discarding the skin.

6 Use a fork or potato masher to mash the eggplant flesh until smooth.

7 Add the olive oil, garlic, tahini, lemon juice, cumin, and paprika to the mashed eggplant. Stir well to combine, ensuring that all ingredients are evenly incorporated and the dip is smooth and creamy. Season with salt and pepper to taste. Refrigerate covered for at least 30 minutes to allow the flavors to set.

8 If desired, garnish the eggplant dip with chopped fresh parsley, a sprinkle of smoked paprika, and a drizzle of extra-virgin olive oil for presentation.

9 Serve the dip with gluten-free crackers, gluten-free bread, or sliced vegetables for dipping.

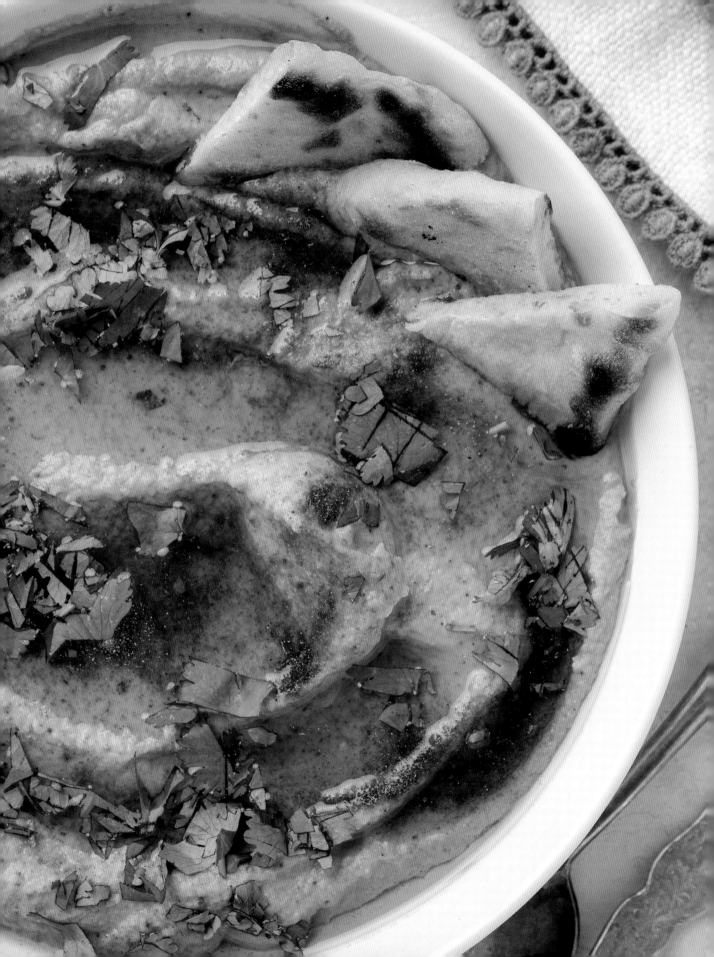

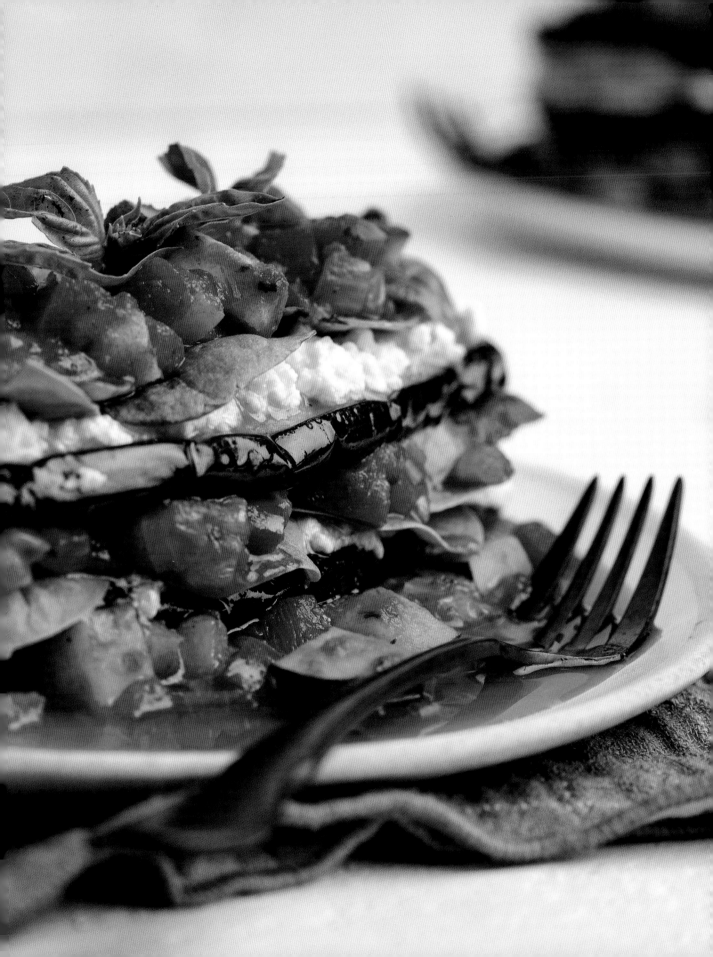

EGGPLANT LASAGNA STACK

Tom: If you can read this description without your mouth watering, I grant you permission to skip this recipe. Slices of roasted eggplant are used to layer this lasagna with their rich, earthy flavor and crisp texture. The filling combines sautéed vegetables—onion, garlic, bell peppers, zucchini, and mushrooms—enhanced with oregano and basil, all simmered in marinara sauce for depth. Creamy ricotta cheese and spinach leaves are spread between each layer. Topped with fresh basil, this lasagna stack promises both visual appeal and a comforting, wholesome meal in every bite.

SERVINGS: 4	PREP TIME: 20 MINUTES	TOTAL TIME: 40 MINUTES

2 medium eggplants
2 tablespoons olive oil, divided
Salt and pepper, to taste
1 white onion, finely chopped
3 garlic cloves, minced

1 red bell pepper, diced
1 yellow bell pepper, diced
1 zucchini, diced
1 cup baby bella mushrooms, sliced
1 teaspoon dried oregano
1 teaspoon dried basil

1 (24-ounce/680g) jar marinara sauce, gluten-free and dairy-free
1 cup dairy-free ricotta cheese, almond- or tofu-based
3–4 cups fresh spinach leaves
Fresh basil leaves, optional

1 Preheat the oven to 400°F (200°C).

2 Wash the eggplant, cut off the stem and the bottom tip. Using a mandoline, slice the eggplant lengthwise into ¼-inch (6mm) planks. Lay the slices out on a baking sheet lined with parchment paper.

3 Brush both sides of the eggplant slices with 1 tablespoon olive oil and season with salt and pepper. Roast for about 15 to 20 minutes or until the slices are tender and slightly browned. Remove from the oven and set aside to cool.

4 While the eggplant is roasting, heat the remaining 1 tablespoon of olive oil in a large skillet over medium heat. Add the onion and garlic, and sauté until softened and fragrant, about 3 to 4 minutes.

5 Add the red and yellow bell peppers, zucchini, and mushrooms to the skillet. Cook, stirring occasionally, until the vegetables are tender, about 5 to 6 minutes. Add the oregano and basil. Season with salt and pepper to taste.

6 Pour the marinara sauce into the skillet with the cooked vegetables. Stir well to combine, then reduce the heat to low and let the sauce simmer for about 5 minutes.

7 To assemble the lasagna, start by spreading a thin layer of marinara-vegetable mixture on the bottom of a serving plate. Place one of the roasted eggplant slices on top of the sauce. The goal is to reconstruct the eggplants back whole but with the layers between it.

8 Spoon 2 to 3 tablespoons of dairy-free ricotta cheese over the eggplant slice, spreading it out evenly with a spatula. Top with 4 to 5 fresh spinach leaves and 23 tablespoons of the marinara.

9 Repeat the layers, alternating between roasted eggplant slices, dairy-free ricotta cheese, spinach leaves, and marinara sauce until you have built one eggplant whole. Finish with a layer of marinara sauce over the top. Repeat the steps with the second eggplant and remaining ricotta, spinach, and marinara.

10 Garnish the lasagna with fresh basil leaves, if using, and serve immediately.

COCONUT CURRY CHICKEN & VEGETABLES

Rachael: The longest period of pregnancy to me is always weeks 20 through 30, but once you've hit 30 weeks, time seems to fly. Suddenly, it feels like you have all the time in the world and none at all. Between baby showers, designing a nursery, and getting your hospital bag ready, the to-do list can start to feel heavy. Sometimes, your mind is in a million places, and you forget to celebrate exactly where you are right now. So tonight, I want you to sit down and celebrate your 30-week milestone with some coconut curry chicken. Coconut curry was a biweekly staple for me, so I thought it would be a fun milestone meal.

SERVINGS: 2–3	PREP TIME: 10 MINUTES	TOTAL TIME: 35–40 MINUTES

1 pound (450g) boneless, skinless chicken breasts or thighs, cut into bite-size pieces
Salt and pepper, to taste
1 tablespoon coconut oil or olive oil
1 white onion, diced
3 garlic cloves, minced
1 tablespoon grated fresh ginger
2 tablespoons curry powder
1 teaspoon ground turmeric
1 (14-ounce/397g) can coconut milk
1 cup chicken broth
Juice of 1 lime
1 red or orange bell pepper cut into strips
4 ounces (113g) sugar snap peas
2 cups chopped fresh broccoli
1 cup shredded carrots

SERVING OPTIONS
Fresh cilantro, for garnish
Cooked rice
Cooked quinoa
Cooked rice noodles

1 Season the chicken pieces evenly with salt and pepper.

2 In a large skillet or pot, heat the coconut oil over medium heat.

3 Add the onion and cook until softened, about 3 to 4 minutes.

4 Stir in the garlic and ginger, and cook for an additional 1 to 2 minutes until fragrant.

5 Add the curry powder and ground turmeric to the skillet, stirring well to coat the onion mixture.

6 Add the seasoned chicken pieces to the skillet and cook until browned on all sides, about 5 to 6 minutes.

7 Pour in the coconut milk, chicken broth, and lime juice, stirring to combine.

8 Bring the mixture to a simmer, then reduce the heat to low, and let it cook for 10 minutes, allowing the flavors to meld and the chicken to cook through.

9 Stir in the bell pepper, sugar snap peas, broccoli, and carrots, and cook for an additional 5 to 7 minutes or until the vegetables are tender and the chicken is cooked through.

10 Taste the curry and adjust the seasoning with salt and pepper as needed.

11 Serve hot garnished with fresh cilantro, alongside cooked rice, quinoa, or rice noodles, if desired.

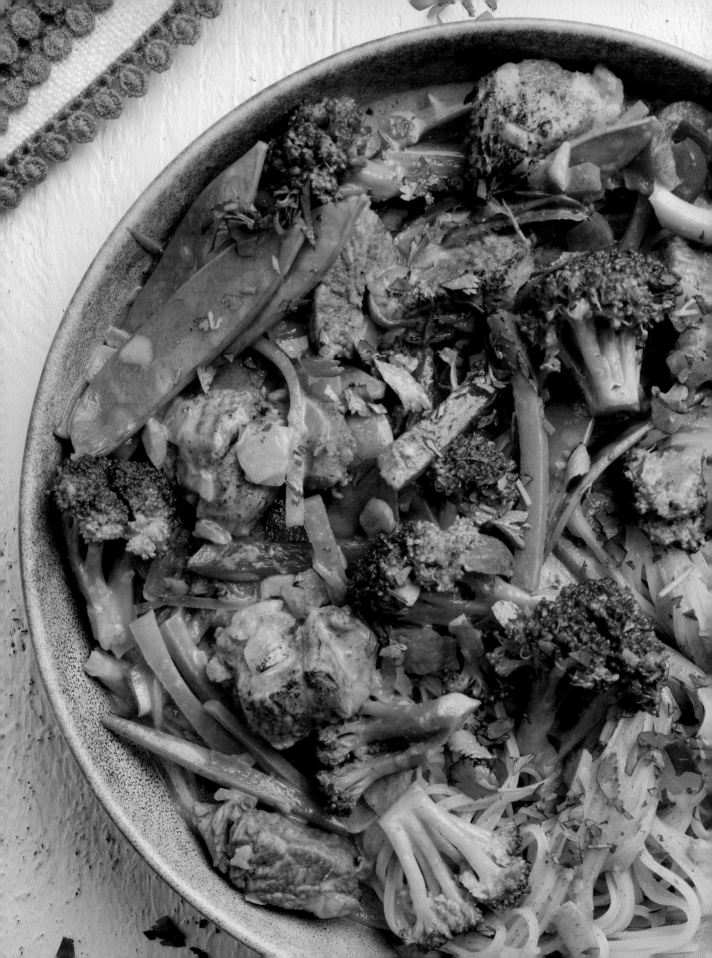

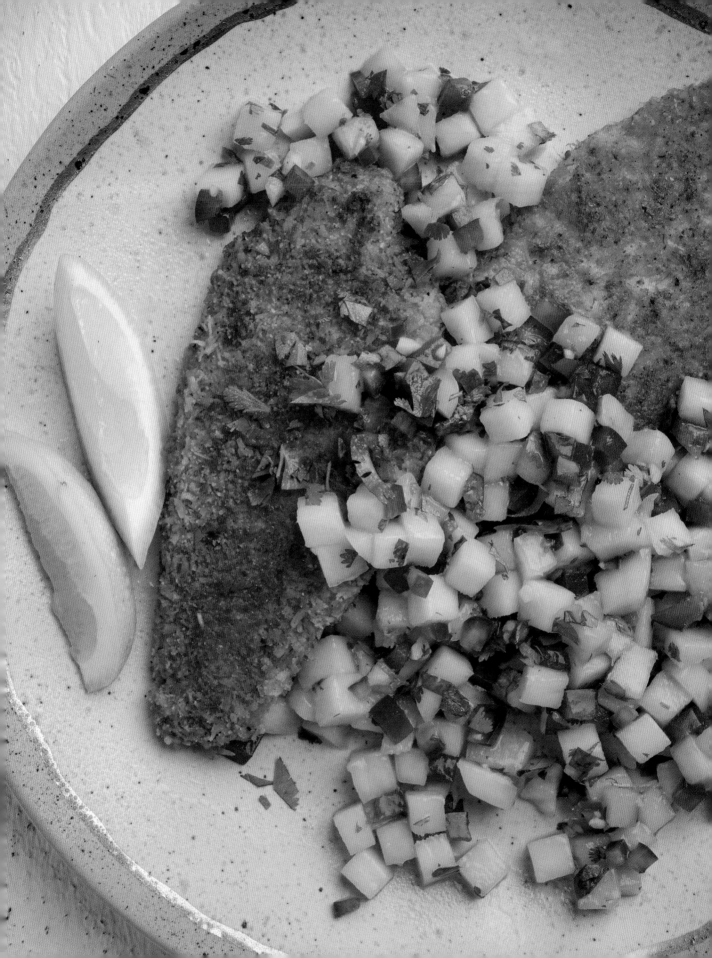

COCONUT-CRUSTED SEAFOOD

WITH MANGO SALSA

Rachael: I had a love-hate relationship with fish during my pregnancies. Some days, the thought of fish would turn my stomach, but other days, I craved it. The days I craved it, I wanted it coconut crusted with some sort of salsa. You can follow this recipe using cod, grouper, halibut, or shrimp. The whitefish are mild in taste, so the flavors of the coconut and mango will pop through!

SERVINGS: 2–4	PREP TIME: 15 MINUTES	TOTAL TIME: 25 MINUTES

½ cup unsweetened shredded coconut

¼ cup rice flour or coconut flour

¼ teaspoon garlic powder

¼ teaspoon paprika

¼ teaspoon salt, adjust to taste

¼ teaspoon black pepper, adjust to taste

1 pound (450g) whitefish fillets or large shrimp, peeled and deveined

2 large eggs, beaten

2 tablespoons coconut oil or olive oil

Chopped fresh cilantro or parsley

Lemon wedges, optional

FOR THE MANGO SALSA

1 large ripe mango, peeled and diced

Juice of 1 lime

¼ red bell pepper, finely diced

1 garlic clove, minced

½ jalapeño, ribs and seeds removed, minced

¼ cup chopped cilantro

¼ teaspoon kosher salt

1 **Prepare the mango salsa.** Combine all the ingredients in a medium bowl and gently toss to combine. (Adjust the amount of jalapeño to suit your taste.) Cover and refrigerate until ready to serve.

2 In a shallow dish, combine the shredded coconut, flour, garlic powder, paprika, salt, and black pepper. Mix well to combine.

3 Pat the fish fillets dry with paper towels and then season with salt and pepper.

4 Add the beaten eggs to a medium bowl and dip each fillet into the eggs, then coat it evenly with the flour mixture, pressing gently to adhere.

5 In a large skillet, heat the coconut oil over medium heat.

6 Once the oil is hot, add the coated fish fillets to the skillet in a single layer, making sure not to overcrowd the pan.

7 Cook the fish fillets for 3 to 4 minutes per side or until golden brown and cooked through. If using shrimp, cook for 2 to 3 minutes per side, until opaque and crispy.

8 Remove the coconut-crusted fish from the skillet and transfer to a serving platter.

9 Garnish with fresh cilantro or parsley and serve with lemon wedges on the side, if desired.

PIÑA COLADA

Rachael: If you like piña coladas and getting caught in the rain, then you will love this recipe. For both of my pregnancies, we just so happened to be on a beach trip in Florida when the babies were the size of a coconut, so Tom made to-go cups of this recipe to enjoy with our toes in the sand. If you haven't planned a beach trip in a while, this is your sign to put one on the calendar. It could be a goal that is weeks, months, or even a year from now. That is, unless you hate the beach, then by all means you do you instead.

SERVINGS: 2	PREP TIME: 10 MINUTES	TOTAL TIME: 10 MINUTES

1 cup fresh pineapple chunks
½ cup full-fat coconut milk
¼ cup coconut cream
1 tablespoon honey
Juice of 1 lime
1 cup ice cubes

SERVING OPTIONS
Pineapple wedges
Pitted maraschino cherries
Mini umbrellas

1 In a blender, combine the fresh pineapple chunks, coconut milk, coconut cream, honey, lime juice, and ice cubes.

2 Blend on high speed until smooth and creamy.

3 Taste the piña colada and adjust the sweetness by adding more honey if needed.

4 To serve, pour the piña colada into glasses and garnish each glass with a pineapple wedge, cherry, and paper umbrella if desired.

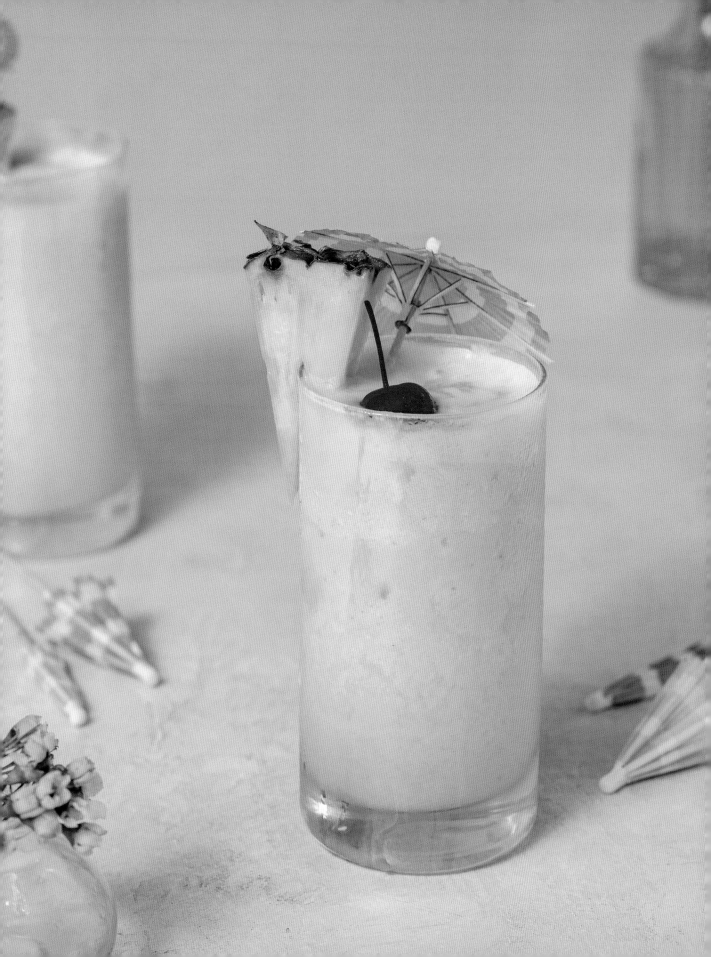

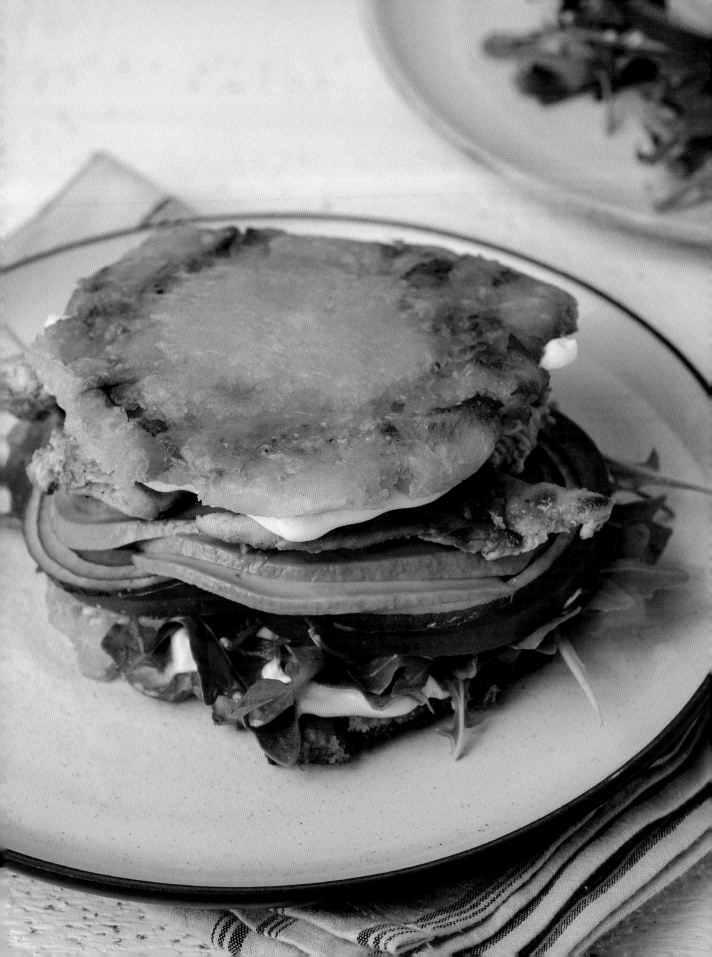

JIBARITO CHICKEN SANDWICH
WITH GARLIC SAUCE

Rachael: Chances are you shared with family or friends that you were pregnant with the "bun in the oven" idiom. This week's recipe is all about that bun in the oven, but with the most delicious "bun" you've ever tasted. Instead of using bread, a jibarito uses tostones (fried plantain slices) as the bun. Filled with meat and a special garlic sauce and then topped with lettuce and tomato, I promise you won't find another sandwich like it.

SERVINGS: 3–4	PREP TIME: 1 HOUR	TOTAL TIME: 1 HOUR 20 MINUTES OR OVERNIGHT TO MARINATE

2 unripe yellow plantains, peeled and cut into 1-inch (2.5cm) pieces (about 3–4 per plantain)

¼ cup plus 1 tablespoon olive oil, divided

Pinch of flaky salt

1 cup arugula

1 ripe avocado, sliced

1 tomato sliced

¼ cup thinly sliced red onion

FOR THE MARINATED CHICKEN

1 tablespoon olive oil

2 garlic cloves, minced

1 teaspoon ground cumin

1 teaspoon smoked paprika

Juice of 1 lime

Salt and pepper, to taste

1 pound (450g) boneless, skinless chicken breasts or thighs, thinly sliced

FOR THE GARLIC SAUCE

¾ cup mayonnaise

3 garlic cloves, minced

1 tablespoon lemon juice

½ teaspoon salt

½ teaspoon pepper

1 **Prepare the marinated chicken.** In a large zipper-lock bag or lidded bowl, combine 1 tablespoon olive oil, 2 minced garlic cloves, cumin, paprika, lime juice, and salt and pepper, to taste. Add the chicken to the bag and refrigerate for at least 1 hour or up to overnight.

2 **Prepare the garlic sauce.** Combine all the garlic sauce ingredients in a small bowl, cover and refrigerate for at least 1 hour or up to overnight.

3 **Make the jibaritos.** In a large pot, bring 4 quarts (4L) of water to a boil over high heat. Add the plantain pieces and cook for 4 to 6 minutes. The yellow color will brighten slightly and the plantains will soften.

4 Remove the plantain pieces and place them between sheets of parchment paper. Flatten the pieces, one at a time, using a flat-bottomed pot or plate to press them. If they crumble, they need more time in the water.

5 In a medium skillet, heat ¼ cup olive oil over medium-high heat to shallow-fry the plantains. Add the flattened plantains in batches, cooking for 2 to 3 minutes on each side, until golden brown and slightly caramelized. Use additional olive oil if needed. Remove and transfer to a plate lined with a paper towel. Sprinkle with flaky salt.

6 In another large skillet, heat 1 tablespoon olive oil over medium-high heat. Remove the chicken from the marinade and place it in the skillet. Feel free to pour the marinade in with the chicken. Sauté for 10 to 12 minutes, stirring and turning occasionally until the chicken is fully cooked and slightly browned.

7 To assemble, lay out two plantain buns for each jibarito. Spread the insides of the buns with garlic sauce. Add arugula, avocado, tomato, onion, and chicken. Top with the second bun, garlic side down.

— week 31 —

BROILED PLANTAIN ICE CREAM SPLIT

Tom: Elevate a classic banana split by substituting ripe plantains, broiled to enhance their natural sweetness, and celebrate another milestone in your pregnancy with this fun dessert! I vividly remember sitting on the couch, this week in the pregnancy, running through all the things we wished we had done, documented, or needed to complete ASAP. Join us if you're in that boat, or applaud yourself if you're ahead of your plans—it's all part of the journey. Either way, enjoy this treat as a sweet reward amidst the excitement and preparations for the new arrival.

SERVINGS: 2–4	**PREP TIME:** 10 MINUTES	**TOTAL TIME:** 20 MINUTES

2 ripe plantains, peeled and halved lengthwise

2 tablespoons melted coconut oil or butter, divided

1 tablespoon honey or maple syrup

½ teaspoon ground cinnamon

¼ teaspoon ground allspice

¼ teaspoon ground nutmeg

Pinch of salt

¼ cup chopped nuts, such as almonds, walnuts, or pecans

1 pint vanilla bean dairy-free ice cream or ice cream of choice

SERVING OPTIONS

Cherries

Sprinkles

Chocolate Syrup

1 Preheat the broiler to high with an oven rack as close to the heating element as possible.

2 Place the halved plantains cut side down on a baking sheet lined with foil. Brush the tops with 1 tablespoon melted coconut oil.

3 Broil the top side of the plantains for 3 to 4 minutes until they start to brown. Remove from the oven and allow to cool.

4 In a small bowl, combine the remaining 1 tablespoon melted coconut oil, honey, cinnamon, allspice, nutmeg, and salt.

5 Flip the cooled plantains over and brush the spice mixture over the cut side of each plantain half.

6 Place the baking sheet back under the broiler and broil for 3 to 4 minutes or until the tops of the plantains are caramelized and golden brown. Keep a close eye on them to prevent burning.

7 Remove the baking sheet from the broiler and sprinkle chopped nuts over the caramelized plantains.

8 Transfer the broiled plantain halves to serving plates. Top each plantain with ice cream and any desired toppings of choice, like cherries, sprinkles, and chocolate syrup, and serve.

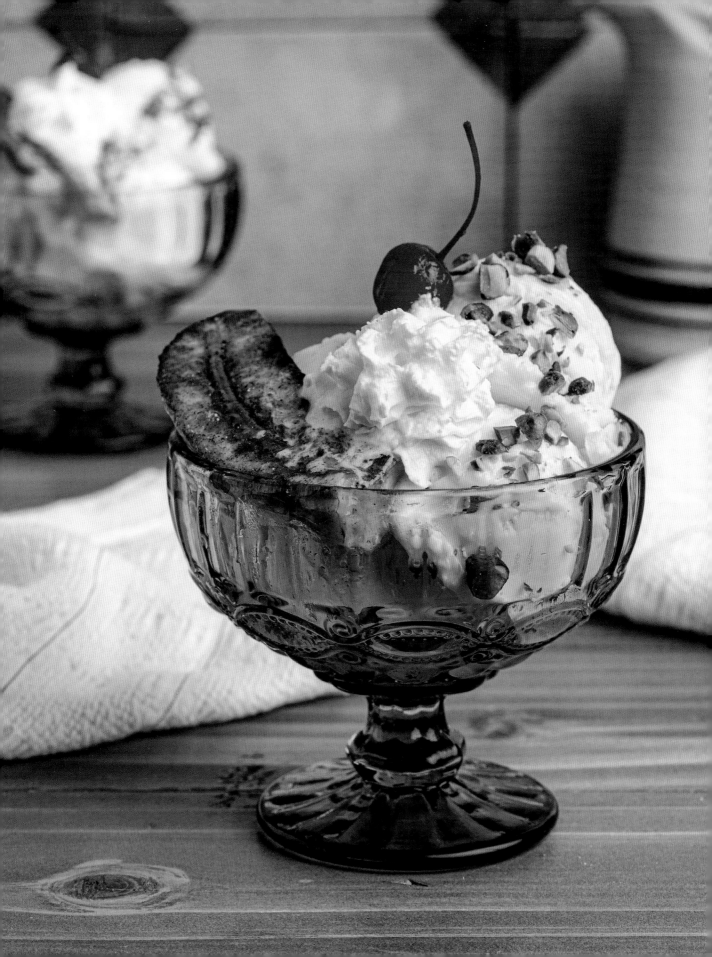

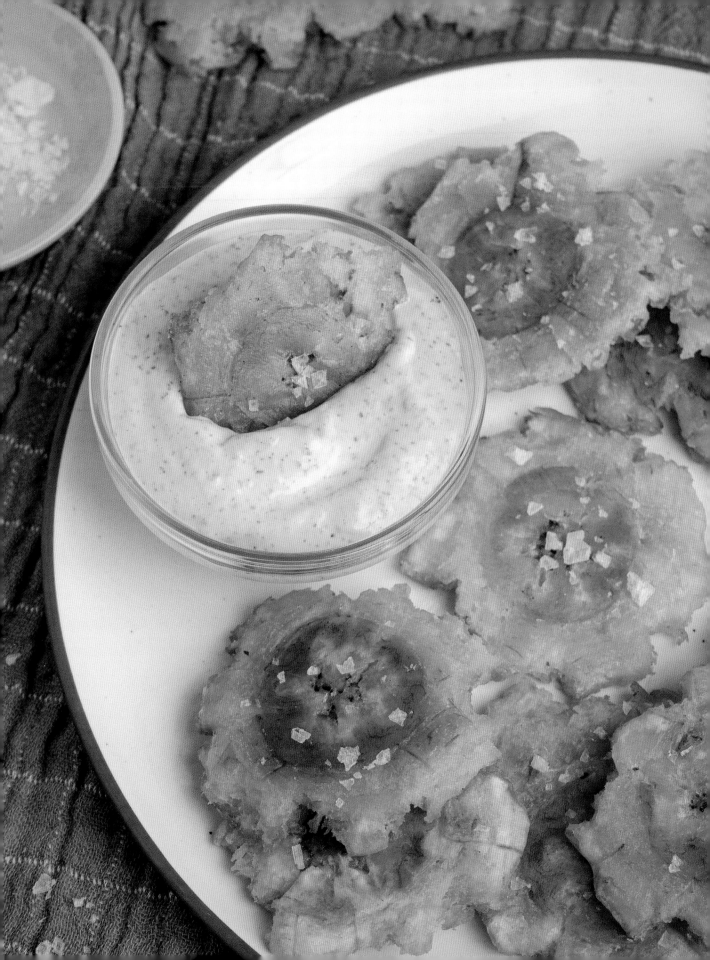

— week 31 —

TOSTONES
WITH HERB DIPPING SAUCE

Rachael: If you have been craving chips this pregnancy, let me turn you on to **tostones**. If you haven't heard of them already, they are made from green plantains (not to be confused with bananas) and are crispy in texture on the outside and soft on the inside. Sprinkled with some salt and paired with a dipping sauce, you will quickly fall in love with this Puerto Rican dish.

SERVINGS: 2–3	PREP TIME: 10 MINUTES	TOTAL TIME: 30 MINUTES

1 cup olive oil, for frying
2 green plantains, peeled and cut into
  1-inch (2.5cm) slices
Pinch of flaky salt

FOR THE HERB DIPPING SAUCE
1 cup mayonnaise
2 tablespoons chopped fresh cilantro
2 tablespoons chopped fresh parsley
1 tablespoon chopped fresh chives
Zest of 1 lime
1 tablespoon lime juice
1 garlic clove, grated
Salt and pepper, to taste

1 Heat the olive oil in a large skillet over medium heat until it reaches about 350°F (180°C).

2 Place the plantain slices in the oil and fry in batches until golden brown, about 3 minutes each side. Be careful not to overfill the skillet. Remove and transfer to a wire rack to cool. Keep the oil at around 350°F (180°C) for the second fry.

3 Place the plantain slices between sheets of parchment paper. Flatten the pieces, one at a time, using a flat pot or plate to press them down.

4 Place the flattened plantains back into the oil to cook for about 1 minute each side until golden and crispy.

5 Remove the tostones from the oil using a slotted spoon and transfer them to a paper towel–lined plate to drain excess oil. Sprinkle them with flaky salt.

6 **Prepare the herb dipping sauce.** In a small bowl, add all the herb dipping sauce ingredients and stir well to combine. Season with salt and pepper to taste. This can also be blended if you prefer a smoother consistency.

7 Serve the plantains hot alongside the herb dipping sauce and enjoy.

CUBAN SLAW

Rachael: This Cuban slaw was inspired by a time when we were feeding thousands of college students by the masses. Sutton was the size of a cabbage, and we were hosting our first-ever year-end college party. These parties were a way for students in our area to come together for free food, community, and one last hurrah before finals and summer break. Because it was a pig roast, a slaw seemed like a fitting side to incorporate cabbage, but with Tom, everything has a twist. I promise, you've never had a slaw like this before, and your tastebuds will be pleasantly surprised.

SERVINGS: 4	PREP TIME: 15 MINUTES	TOTAL TIME: 1 HOUR

1 cup diced sweet or dill pickles with juice
1 cup sliced pickled banana peppers with juice
1–2 medium jalapeños, thinly sliced
½ cup finely diced cilantro
¼ head green cabbage, shredded
½ head red cabbage, shredded
1 carrot, shredded

FOR THE SAUCE
Juice of 2 oranges
Juice of ½ lime
¼ cup red wine vinegar
2 garlic cloves, minced
2 tablespoons Dijon mustard
1 tablespoon stone-ground mustard
1 tablespoon agave syrup
¼ cup avocado oil or olive oil
1 teaspoon dried oregano
½ teaspoon ground cumin
Salt and pepper, to taste
¾ cup mayonnaise, optional

1 **Make the sauce.** Add all the sauce ingredients to a medium bowl and mix well to combine. Include mayonnaise for a creamier sauce. Place the sauce in the fridge for at least 30 minutes to chill.

2 **Prepare the slaw.** Toss the pickles, banana peppers, jalapeños, cilantro, cabbage, and carrot together in a separate medium bowl to combine.

3 Remove the chilled sauce from the fridge and add it to the combined slaw ingredients. Mix well, coating the slaw evenly, and place the bowl back in the fridge for at least 15 additional minutes to chill before serving.

Note *Pairs well with the pulled pork sandwiches, tacos, or bowls (page 206) as a side dish or condiment.*

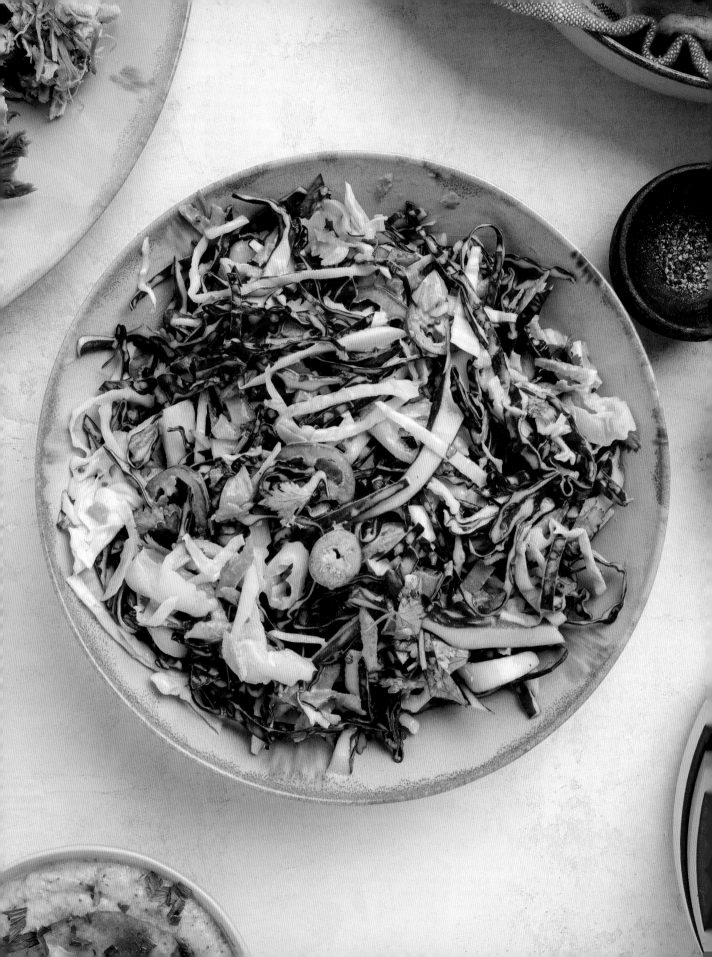

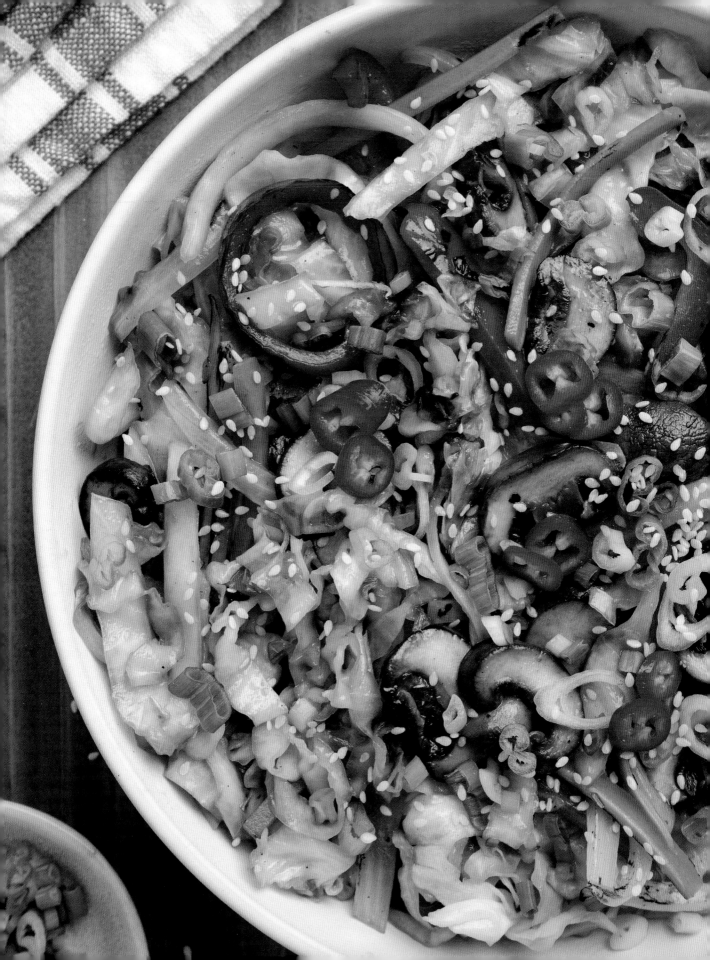

CABBAGE STIR-FRY

Rachael: So often during my pregnancy, I craved vegetables. Something about a big bowl of veggies made me feel like the baby was getting all the proper nutrients needed that day. Stir-fries are a great way to incorporate tons of different vegetables into one dish. In this dish, you will find carrots, bell peppers, mushrooms, and cabbage, of course, all of which contain amazing sources of vitamins and nutrients to help support baby development.

SERVINGS: 4–6	PREP TIME: 10 MINUTES	TOTAL TIME: 30 MINUTES

1 tablespoon olive oil or coconut oil
1 white onion, thinly sliced
2 garlic cloves, minced
1 tablespoon grated ginger
2 carrots, peeled and julienned or thinly sliced
1 red bell pepper, thinly sliced
4 ounces (113g) sliced baby bella mushrooms
1 small head green cabbage, thinly sliced
Salt and pepper to taste

FOR THE SAUCE
2 tablespoons gluten-free tamari or soy sauce
1 tablespoon rice vinegar
1 tablespoon sesame oil
1 tablespoon honey

SERVING OPTIONS
Sesame seeds
Chopped green onions
Sliced fresh red chili pepper

1   **Prepare the sauce.** In a small bowl, whisk together the gluten-free tamari, rice vinegar, sesame oil, and honey. Set aside.

2   **Start the stir-fry.** Heat olive oil in a large skillet or wok over medium-high heat.

3   Add the onion to the skillet and cook for 2 to 3 minutes, until softened.

4   Add the garlic and ginger to the skillet. Cook for about 1 minute, until fragrant.

5   Add the carrots, bell pepper, and mushrooms to the skillet. Cook for another 3 to 4 minutes, until the vegetables are slightly tender but still crisp. Season with salt and pepper to taste.

6   Add the cabbage to the skillet. Stir well to combine with the other vegetables.

7   Cook the stir-fry for 5 to 6 minutes, stirring frequently, until the cabbage is wilted but still slightly crisp.

8   Pour the prepared stir-fry sauce over the vegetables in the skillet.

9   Stir well to coat all the vegetables evenly with the sauce.

10   Continue to cook for another 2 to 3 minutes, until the sauce has thickened slightly and coats the vegetables.

11   Remove the skillet from heat and transfer the stir-fry to serving plates.

12   Garnish with sesame seeds, chopped green onions, and fresh red chili pepper slices, if desired.

STUFFED CABBAGE ROLLS
WITH TOMATO SAUCE

Rachael: Here I am at 32 weeks pregnant, writing you this love letter to say your girl is feeling uncomfortable. I'm trying to fit into clothes that no longer serve me, sleep has become a challenge, and I know these symptoms are only going to progress, so this meal is made to add some comfort back into your life. These stuffed cabbage rolls have a hearty filling that will make you feel cozy and want to savor every bite.

SERVINGS: 4–6	PREP TIME: 15 MINUTES	TOTAL TIME: 1 HOUR 35 MINUTES

1 large head of cabbage, cored
1 tablespoon olive oil
1 yellow onion, finely chopped
2 garlic cloves, minced
2 carrots, peeled and diced
½ sweet potato, peeled and diced
1 pound (450g) lean ground turkey or beef
1 cup cooked quinoa or cauliflower rice
1 teaspoon dried oregano
1 teaspoon dried basil
Salt and pepper, to taste

FOR THE TOMATO SAUCE
2 (14-ounce/397g) cans crushed tomatoes with juice
2 tablespoons tomato paste
2 teaspoons dried oregano
2 teaspoons dried basil
Salt and pepper, to taste

1 Bring a large pot of water to a boil. Carefully remove any damaged outer leaves from the cabbage.

2 Carefully place the whole cabbage head in the boiling water and cook for 5 to 7 minutes or until the outer leaves are softened and easily peel off.

3 Remove the cabbage from the water and carefully peel off 12 to 15 large leaves. Set aside to cool.

4 **Prepare the tomato sauce.** In a small saucepan, combine the crushed tomatoes, tomato paste, 2 teaspoons oregano, 2 teaspoons basil, and season to taste with salt and pepper.

5 Cook over medium heat, stirring occasionally, for 5 to 7 minutes to allow the flavors to come together. Remove from the heat and set aside.

6 **Make the cabbage-roll filling.** In a large skillet, heat olive oil over medium heat.

7 Add the onion and garlic to the skillet. Cook until softened and fragrant, about 2 minutes. Add the carrots and sweet potato and cook for 5 more minutes.

8 Add the ground turkey to the skillet and adjust the heat to medium high. Cook until browned, about 8 to 10 minutes, breaking up the meat with a spoon as it cooks.

9 Stir in the cooked quinoa, ½ cup of the fresh-made tomato sauce, 1 teaspoon oregano, 1 teaspoon basil, and season to taste with salt and pepper. Cook for an additional 2 to 3 minutes, until heated through.

10 **Assemble and bake the stuffed cabbage rolls.** Preheat the oven to 375°F (190°C).

11 Place about ¼ cup of the filling mixture onto each cooled cabbage leaf, near the stem end.

12 Roll up the cabbage leaf, tucking in the sides as you go, to encase the filling. Repeat with the remaining cabbage leaves, filling each. As you assemble them, place the cabbage rolls seam side down in a 9x13-inch (23x33cm) baking dish.

13 Pour the remaining fresh-made tomato sauce over the cabbage rolls, covering them evenly.

14 Cover the baking dish with aluminum foil and bake for 45 to 50 minutes or until the cabbage rolls are cooked through and tender.

15 Plate the cabbage rolls, top with tomato sauce from the pan, and enjoy!

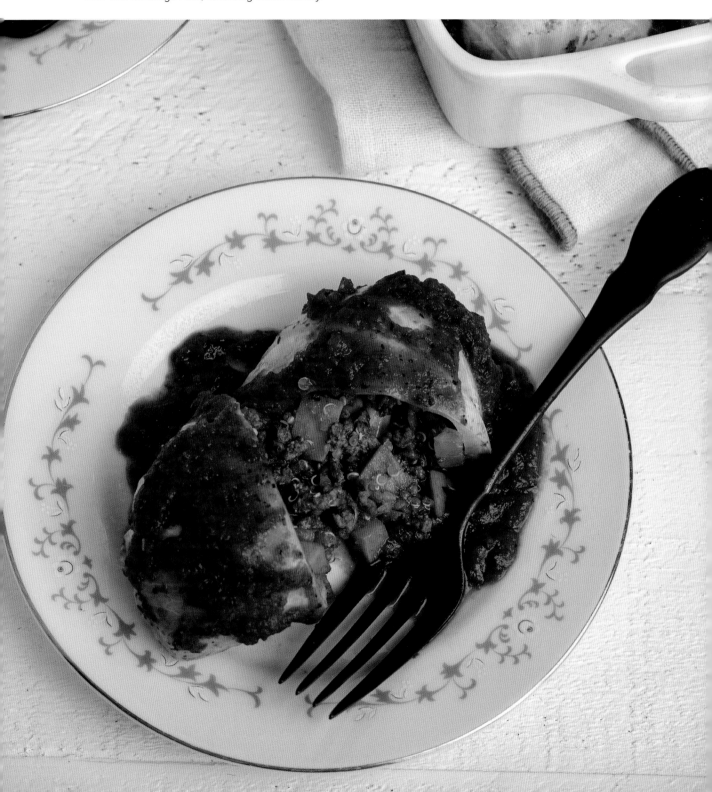

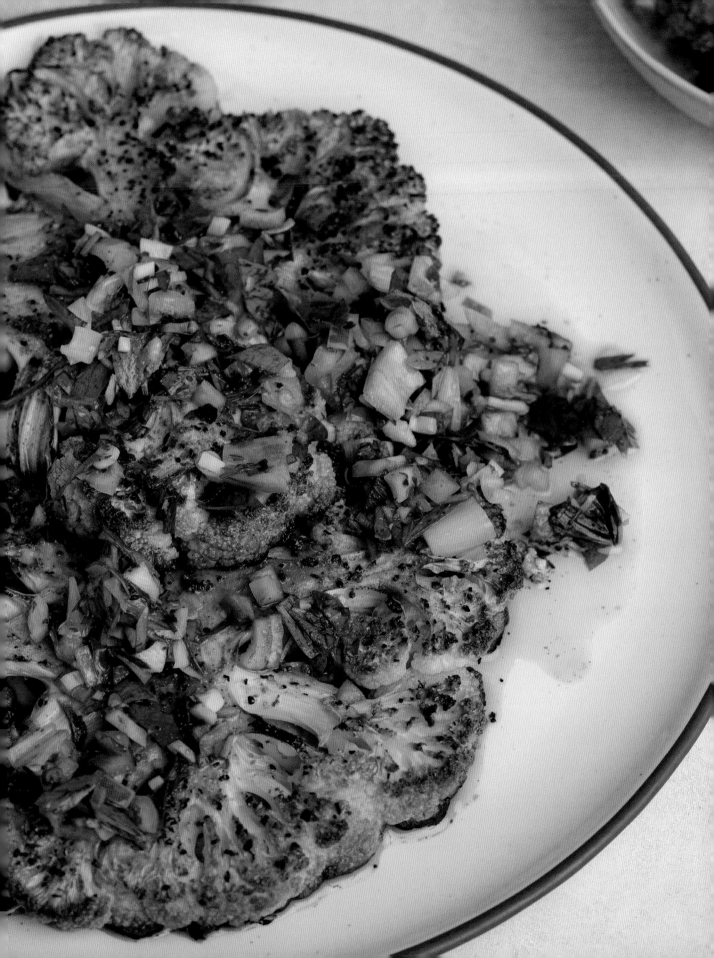

CAULIFLOWER STEAK
WITH CHIMICHURRI

Rachael: Can you believe your baby is the size of a head of cauliflower? The human body and what it is capable of is simply amazing. To stay on theme of "anything is possible," we are transforming cauliflower into steak this week. The cauliflower will be cut, seared, and topped with a chimichurri sauce. My favorite part of this recipe is the sauce, and I know you will be finding yourself using it for other dishes in the future.

SERVINGS: 4	PREP TIME: 5 MINUTES	TOTAL TIME: 30 MINUTES

1 large cauliflower head
1 teaspoon salt
1 teaspoon black pepper
1 teaspoon garlic powder
1 teaspoon smoked paprika
2 tablespoons olive oil

FOR THE CHIMICHURRI
1 cup packed fresh flat-leaf or
   Italian parsley leaves
4 garlic cloves, peeled
¼ cup red wine vinegar
½ teaspoon fine sea salt
½ teaspoon red pepper flakes
½ cup finely chopped shallot
½ cup extra-virgin olive oil

Note *Customize this recipe by adding your favorite herbs or spices to the cauliflower steaks before roasting. You can also serve this dish topped with cooked eggs for extra protein or with a side of avocado slices or a simple green salad for added freshness.*

1 **Make the chimichurri.** Add the parsley, garlic, red wine vinegar, salt, red pepper flakes, and shallot to a food processor or blender. Pulse a few times. Slowly pour ½ cup of extra-virgin olive oil into the blender, while pulsing a few more times, until the chimichurri is chopped, but not mushy. Adjust the salt and red pepper flakes to your taste.

2 **Prepare the cauliflower.** Preheat the oven to 400°F (200°C).

3 Remove the outer leaves from the cauliflower head and trim the stem, leaving the core intact.

4 Place the cauliflower upright on a cutting board and slice it into 1-inch-thick (2.5cm) "steaks," starting from the center and working your way out. You should get about four steaks from one cauliflower head, depending on its size.

5 Combine the salt, pepper, garlic powder, and smoked paprika in a small bowl. Brush both sides of each cauliflower steak with the 2 tablespoons olive oil and season with the salt, pepper, and garlic powder mix.

6 Place the cauliflower steaks on a baking sheet lined with parchment paper.

7 Roast in the preheated oven for 20 to 25 minutes, flipping halfway through, until the cauliflower is tender and golden brown around the edges.

8 Once the cauliflower steaks are done roasting, transfer them to serving plates. Top the steaks with the chimichurri.

9 If desired, sprinkle the dish with additional chopped fresh flat-leaf parsley and red pepper flakes, for added flavor and color.

CAULIFLOWER CURRY

Rachael: This is our second curry recipe in this book because I love curry and, selfishly, I felt you needed to spend another week enjoying curry as well. There were multiple occasions during my pregnancy in which I craved curry and pizza at the same time. I needed the marriage of red sauce and curry sauce together or I wasn't satisfied. The fact that we don't have an actual curry pizza recipe in this book is criminal. So don't tell Tom, but this is an official hall pass from me for you to order a small pizza to accompany this meal.

SERVINGS: 4–6	PREP TIME: 10 MINUTES	TOTAL TIME: 50 MINUTES

2 tablespoons coconut oil or olive oil
1 yellow onion, finely chopped
3 garlic cloves, minced
1 tablespoon grated fresh ginger
1 teaspoon ground turmeric
1 teaspoon ground cumin
1 teaspoon ground coriander
½ teaspoon ground cinnamon
¼ teaspoon ground cayenne
1 medium cauliflower, cut into florets
1 (14-ounce/397g) can full-fat coconut milk
1 (14-ounce/397g) can diced tomatoes
1 cup vegetable broth
2 cups fresh baby spinach or chopped kale
Salt and pepper, to taste

SERVING OPTIONS
Chopped fresh cilantro
Cooked rice or quinoa

1 In a large skillet or pot, heat the coconut oil over medium heat.

2 Add the onion, garlic, and ginger. Sauté until softened and fragrant, about 3 to 4 minutes.

3 Add the turmeric, cumin, coriander, cinnamon, and cayenne to the skillet. Stir well to combine with the onion mixture. Cook for an additional 1 to 2 minutes to toast the spices.

4 Add the cauliflower florets to the skillet and stir to coat with the spice mixture.

5 Cook for 5 to 7 minutes, stirring occasionally, until the cauliflower starts to soften.

6 Pour in the coconut milk, diced tomatoes with the juice, and vegetable broth. Stir well to combine. Season with salt and pepper to taste.

7 Bring the mixture to a simmer, then reduce the heat to low. Cover and let it simmer for 15 to 20 minutes, until the cauliflower is tender.

8 Stir in the baby spinach. Cook for an additional 2 to 3 minutes, until the greens are wilted.

9 Taste the curry and season with additional salt and pepper, to taste.

10 Serve the cauliflower curry hot; pour over cooked rice and garnish with cilantro, if desired.

Notes *Feel free to adjust the spices and seasonings according to your taste preferences. If you don't have all the spices on hand, a curry powder seasoning blend also works nicely for this recipe. You can also add other vegetables, such as bell peppers, carrots, or peas, to the curry for extra flavor and nutrition.*

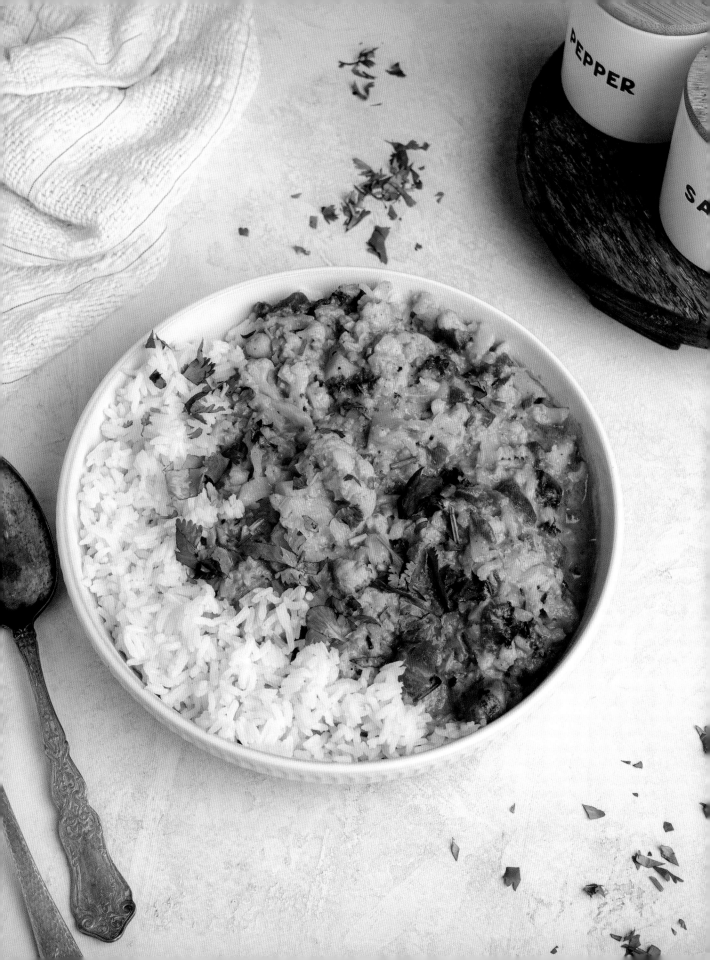

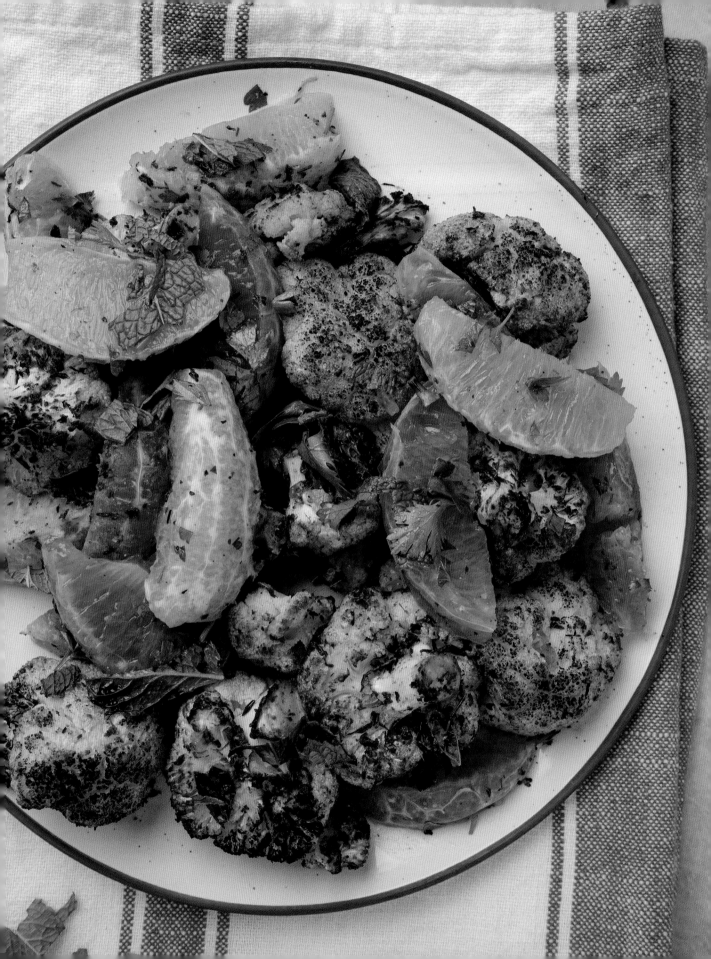

BLACKENED CAULIFLOWER
WITH CITRUS HERB SALAD

Rachael: Has anyone else lost their appetite at this point during pregnancy? For some, the first trimester may have been a grueling time frame with nausea. Then the second trimester arrived and getting your hunger back was like a rainbow after a storm! Some of you may experience another shift in the third trimester where you haven't lost your hunger, but after a few bites you feel full and out of breath, at least that's where I'm at as I write this. This dish is a perfect mix of "I want a few pieces of cauliflower to munch on" paired with "I want to end on a refreshing note," and that's where the citrus herb salad comes in.

SERVINGS: 3–4	**PREP TIME:** 15 MINUTES	**TOTAL TIME:** 40 MINUTES

1 large cauliflower head, cut into florets
2 tablespoons olive oil
1 teaspoon garlic powder
1 teaspoon onion powder
1 teaspoon dried thyme
1 teaspoon smoked paprika
½ teaspoon ground cumin
½ teaspoon dried basil
½ teaspoon dried oregano
¼ teaspoon cayenne
1 teaspoon salt
½ teaspoon black pepper

FOR THE CITRUS HERB SALAD
2 oranges, peeled and segmented
1 grapefruit, peeled and segmented
¼ cup chopped fresh parsley leaves
¼ cup chopped fresh mint leaves
¼ cup chopped fresh cilantro leaves
1 tablespoon extra-virgin olive oil
1 tablespoon freshly squeezed lime
  juice
Salt and pepper, to taste

1 Prepare the blackened cauliflower. Begin by preheating the oven to 425°F (220°C).

2 In a large bowl, toss the cauliflower florets with olive oil until evenly coated.

3 In a separate small bowl, combine the garlic powder, onion powder, thyme, smoked paprika, cumin, basil, oregano, cayenne, salt, and pepper. Mix well.

4 Sprinkle the spice mixture over the cauliflower florets and toss until evenly coated.

5 Spread the cauliflower florets in a single layer on a baking sheet lined with parchment paper.

6 Roast in the preheated oven for 20 to 25 minutes, until the cauliflower is tender and blackened around the edges, flipping the cauliflower halfway through.

7 **Prepare the citrus herb salad.** In a large bowl, combine the orange segments, grapefruit segments, parsley, mint, and cilantro.

8 Drizzle the extra-virgin olive oil and fresh lime juice over the salad.

9 Season with salt and pepper to taste. Toss gently to combine.

10 **Assemble the dish.** Arrange the blackened cauliflower on a serving platter. Spoon the citrus herb salad over the cauliflower. Serve immediately.

Notes   *Feel free to customize the salad with additional herbs or add-ins, such as toasted nuts or seeds, for extra crunch. You can also adjust the level of spiciness of the blackened cauliflower by increasing or decreasing the amount of cayenne to your taste. Should you not have all the spices on hand, a store-bought blackened seasoning blend also works nicely for this recipe.*

— week 34 —

PINEAPPLE WHIP

Rachael: During the summers when I was a kid, my mom loved to find interactive activities to do with us, many of which involved cooking. As a parent, now I get it—you'll do anything to keep your kids entertained, which includes helping make dinner or in this case, dessert. Pineapple whip is incredibly easy to put together with just a few steps, and if you already have kids, this is a fun one to get them involved in. Don't say I never shared any parenting hacks with you.

SERVINGS: 4–6	PREP TIME: 10 MINUTES	TOTAL TIME: 4 HOURS 10 MINUTES OR OVERNIGHT TO FREEZE

1 ripe pineapple; peeled, cored, and diced
½ cup full-fat coconut milk
1½ tablespoons honey
1 teaspoon vanilla extract
Juice of 1 lime, optional
Pinch of salt

SERVING OPTIONS
Fresh pineapple slices
Fresh mint leaves

1 Spread the diced pineapple in a single layer on a baking sheet lined with parchment paper.

2 Place the baking sheet in the freezer and freeze until the pineapple is solid, at least 4 hours or overnight.

3 Once the pineapple is frozen, transfer it to a high-speed blender or food processor. Add the coconut milk, honey, vanilla extract, lime juice (if using), and a pinch of salt.

4 Blend on high until smooth and creamy, scraping down the sides of the blender or food processor as needed. You may need to add a little more coconut milk if the mixture is too thick. Add additional honey to taste.

5 Scoop the pineapple whip into serving bowls or glasses. Garnish with fresh pineapple slices and mint leaves, if desired.

Note *Feel free to customize this recipe by adding other fruits, such as mango or banana, for added flavor variations. You can also experiment with different toppings, such as shredded coconut or chopped nuts, for added texture.*

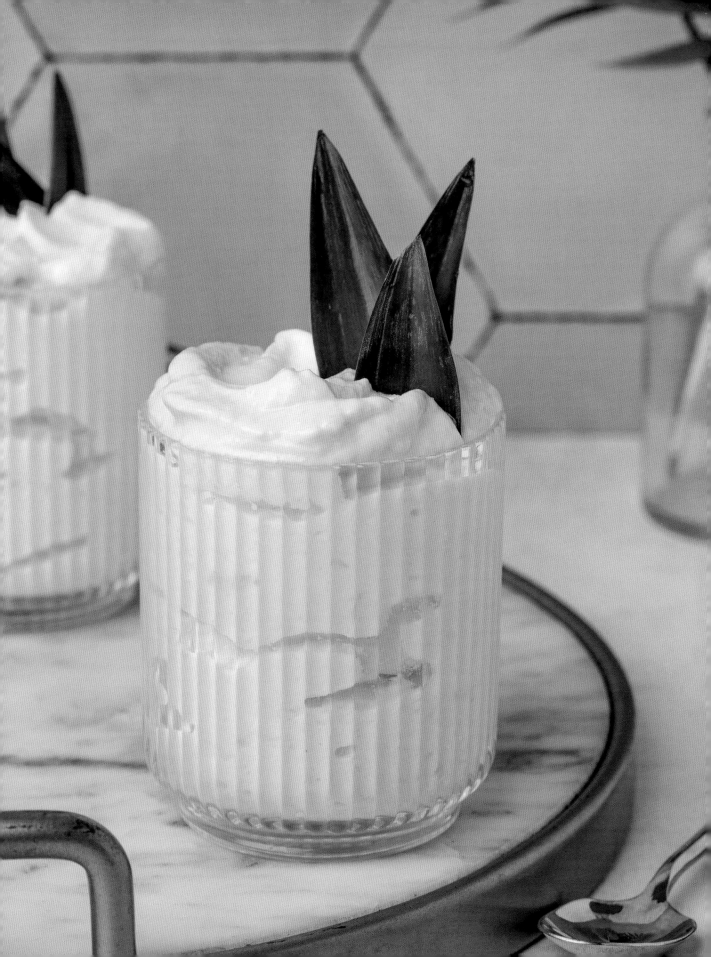

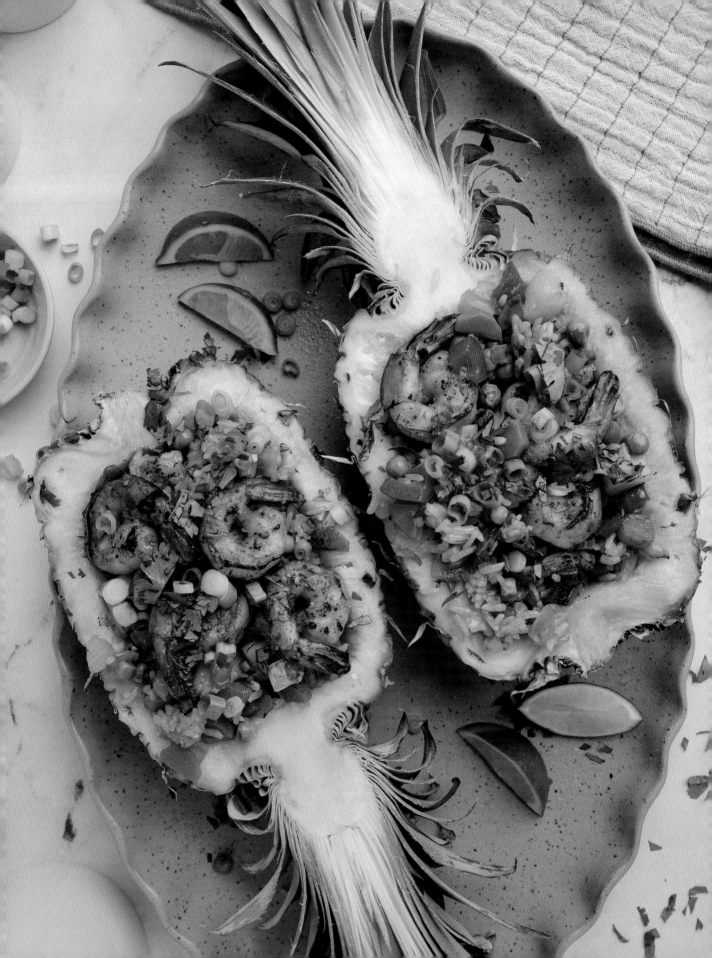

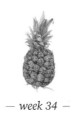

SHRIMP FRIED RICE

IN A PINEAPPLE BOAT

Rachael: Baby update and food descriptions aside, can we all take a moment to appreciate the aesthetics of this photo? Because the shrimp fried rice in a pineapple boat is slayinggg! Pineapple may not belong on pizza (in my humble opinion), but it does belong with fried rice and shrimp, and I think it's kinda mandatory that it be served out of a pineapple (at least once). Please, if you tag us in any meal, can it be this one? We want to repost every bougie pineapple boat pic that comes into our inbox on Instagram or Tiktok (@Rachsullivan__ or @Mealssheeats)!

SERVINGS: 6–8	PREP TIME: 15 MINUTES	TOTAL TIME: 35 MINUTES

1 large ripe pineapple
2 tablespoons coconut oil or olive oil, divided
1 pound (450g) large shrimp, peeled and deveined
Salt and pepper, to taste
1 small white onion, finely chopped

2 garlic cloves, minced
2 carrots, peeled and diced
1 red bell pepper, diced
3 cups cooked rice
1 cup frozen peas, thawed
3 tablespoons gluten-free soy sauce or tamari

2 tablespoons fish sauce, optional
1 tablespoon honey or maple syrup
2 green onions, thinly sliced
Chopped fresh cilantro leaves
Lime wedges

1   Cut the pineapple in half lengthwise. Using a knife and spoon, hollow out both halves of the pineapple to create boats. Reserve the pineapple flesh for the fried rice. Set the pineapple boats aside.

2   Dice the reserved pineapple flesh into small pieces.

3   Heat 1 tablespoon of coconut oil in a large skillet over medium-high heat. Season the shrimp with salt and pepper and add to the skillet. Cook until pink and opaque, about 2 to 3 minutes per side. Remove the shrimp from the skillet and set aside.

4   In the same skillet, heat the remaining 1 tablespoon of coconut oil over medium heat. Add the onion to the skillet. Cook until fragrant and the onion is translucent, about 2 to 3 minutes.

5   Add the garlic, carrots, and red bell pepper to the skillet. Cook until the vegetables are tender, about 5 to 7 minutes.

6   Stir in the cooked rice, diced pineapple, and thawed peas. Cook, stirring occasionally, until the rice is heated through, about 3 to 5 minutes.

7   In a small bowl, whisk together the gluten-free soy sauce, fish sauce (if using), and honey. Pour the sauce over the fried rice in the skillet. Stir to combine, ensuring the rice is evenly coated with the sauce.

8   Return the cooked shrimp to the skillet. Stir to distribute the shrimp throughout the fried rice.

9   Carefully spoon the shrimp fried rice into the hollowed-out pineapple boats. Garnish the shrimp fried rice with thinly sliced green onions and chopped fresh cilantro.

10   Serve hot, with lime wedges on the side for squeezing over the rice.

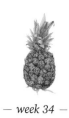

SLOW-COOKER PINEAPPLE PULLED PORK, THREE WAYS

Tom: By this point in both pregnancies, Rachael was moving slowly and getting fatigued quickly. So a slow-cooker recipe that makes a variety of meals—sliders, tacos, or bowls—seemed very fitting. Throw everything into the slow cooker, walk away, and have options for the week. Not to mention, it's delicious and all things sweet, savory, and salty, a favorite combo for us.

SERVINGS: 4–6	**PREP TIME:** 15 MINUTES	**TOTAL TIME:** 4–10 HOURS

1 cup pineapple juice
½ cup gluten-free soy sauce or tamari
¼ cup honey or maple syrup
4 garlic cloves, minced
1 tablespoon grated fresh ginger
1 teaspoon ground cumin
½ teaspoon ground cinnamon
Salt and pepper, to taste
2–3 pound (1361g) pork shoulder or
    pork butt, excess fat trimmed
1 pineapple, peeled, cored, and diced

FOR PULLED-PORK SLIDERS
4-6 gluten-free slider buns
4-6 pineapple rings
Pickled jalapeños, optional
1 cup coleslaw, optional

FOR PULLED-PORK BOWLS
2–3 cups cooked rice
2-3 cups steamed or roasted–
    vegetables
2 tablespoons chopped fresh cilantro
1 small lime, cut in wedges

FOR PULLED-PORK TACOS
8 corn or gluten-free tortillas
1 medium avocado, sliced
1 cup finely shredded cabbage or
    lettuce
2 tablespoons chopped fresh cilantro
1 small lime, cut in wedges
Pickled jalapeños, optional

1 In a large slow cooker, combine the pineapple juice, gluten-free soy sauce, honey, garlic, ginger, cumin, and cinnamon and then season with salt and pepper to taste. Stir to combine.

2 Place the pork shoulder into the slow cooker, ensuring it is well-submerged in the liquid. Add the diced pineapple around the pork.

3 Cover and cook on low heat for 8 to 10 hours or high heat for 4 to 6 hours, until the pork is tender and easily shreds with a fork.

4 Once the pork is cooked, remove it from the slow cooker and transfer it to a cutting board. Use two forks to shred the pork into bite-size pieces. Return the shredded pork to the cooking liquid inside the pot and reduce the heat to low to it keep warm while assembling your sliders, bowls, or tacos.

5 Store leftovers in an airtight container in the refrigerator for up to 4 days.

FOR PULLED-PORK SLIDERS
1 Toast the slider buns if desired.

2 Place a generous portion of pulled pork on each bun and top with sliced pineapple rings, as well as pickled jalapeños and coleslaw, if using. Serve immediately.

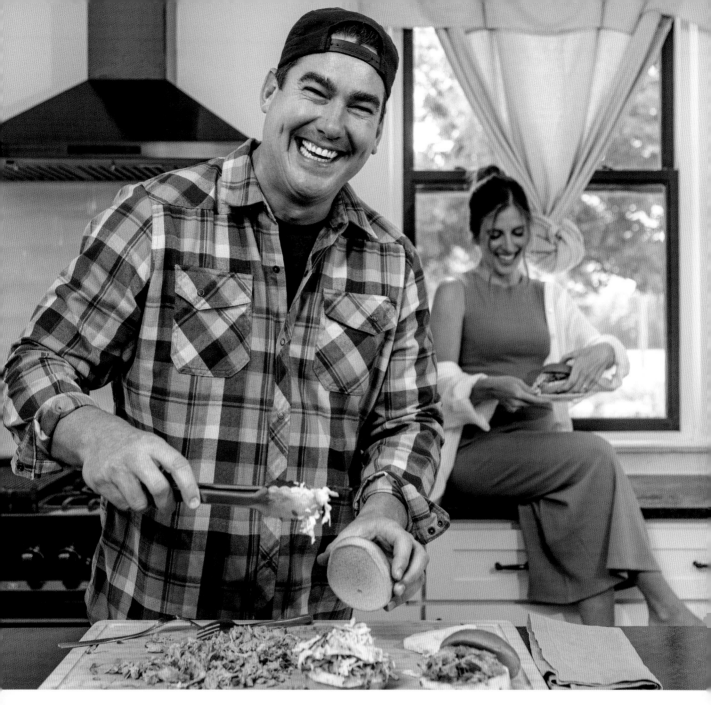

FOR PULLED-PORK BOWLS

1. Divide the cooked rice among serving bowls. Top each bowl of rice with a generous portion of pulled pork and steamed or roasted vegetables of your choice.

2. Garnish with chopped fresh cilantro and squeeze lime wedges over the bowls before serving.

FOR PULLED-PORK TACOS

1. Heat corn tortillas in a skillet or microwave.

2. Fill each tortilla with pulled pork and top with sliced avocado, shredded cabbage, chopped fresh cilantro, and pickled jalapeños if using.

3. Squeeze lime wedges over the tacos and serve immediately.

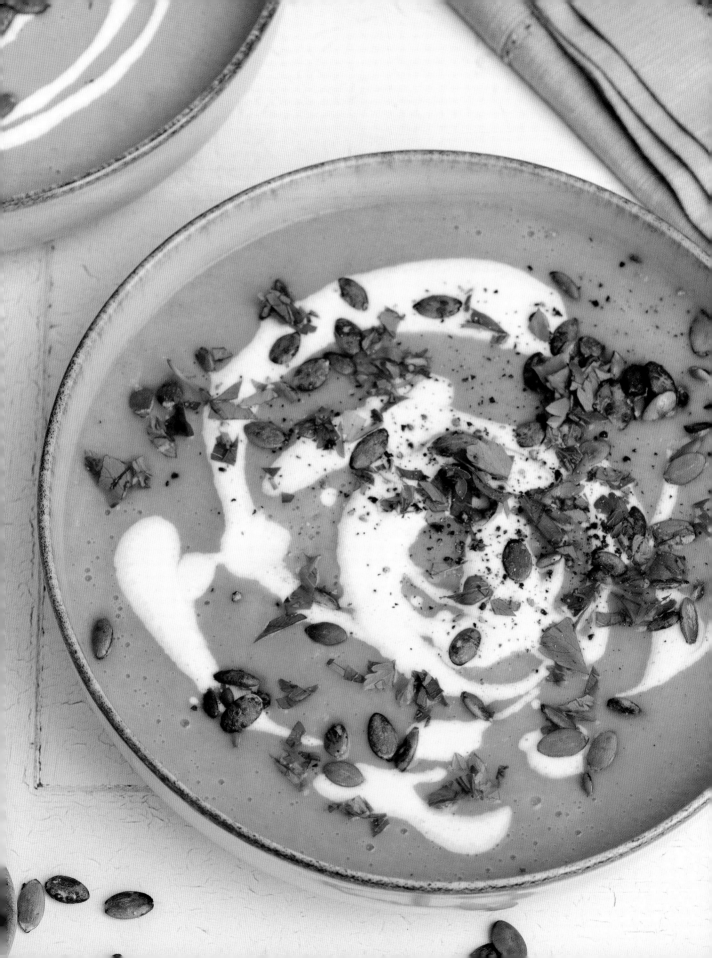

ROASTED BUTTERNUT SQUASH SOUP

Rachael: I have such an obsession with roasted butternut squash soup that I make Tom cook it in bulk to keep in our freezer. (Mainly for when he's out of town, so I will have something to defrost because cooking is not my forte—reheating is.) For some of you, soon, storing things in bulk will become all too familiar with breastfeeding. I could never produce enough milk to keep a frozen stash, but I've seen some of you online with those deep freezers full of stored breast milk, and I always think about how incredible a woman's body is. Whether it's freezing this butternut squash soup or your breast milk, just know someone will have something yummy to eat in the future.

SERVINGS: 3–4	PREP TIME: 10 MINUTES	TOTAL TIME: 40 MINUTES

1 large butternut squash; peeled, seeded, and diced
3 tablespoons olive oil, divided
Salt and pepper, to taste
1 white onion, chopped
2 garlic cloves, minced
2 carrots, peeled and chopped
2 celery stalks, chopped
1 teaspoon ground cumin
½ teaspoon ground cinnamon
¼ teaspoon ground nutmeg
4 cups vegetable broth or chicken broth

SERVING OPTIONS
Plain Greek yogurt or coconut cream
Roasted pumpkin seeds
Chopped fresh herbs

1 Preheat the oven to 400°F (200°C).

2 Place the diced butternut squash on a baking sheet lined with parchment paper. Drizzle with 1½ tablespoons of olive oil and sprinkle with salt and pepper. Toss to coat evenly.

3 Roast the butternut squash in the preheated oven for 25 to 30 minutes, until tender and caramelized.

4 In a large pot, heat the remaining 1½ tablespoons of olive oil over medium heat. Add the onion, garlic, carrots, and celery. Cook until the vegetables are softened, about 5 to 7 minutes.

5 Stir in the cumin, cinnamon, and nutmeg, and cook for another minute until fragrant.

6 Pour in the vegetable broth and bring the mixture to a simmer. Let it simmer for about 10 minutes to allow the flavors to meld.

7 Once the roasted butternut squash is baked, remove it from the oven and add it to the pot with the simmering broth and vegetables. Use an immersion blender or transfer the mixture to a blender in batches, and blend until smooth and creamy. If using a blender, be careful not to overfill it since the mixture is hot and will expand.

8 Season the soup with additional salt and pepper to taste.

9 If desired, garnish each bowl with a dollop of Greek yogurt, roasted pumpkin seeds, and chopped fresh herbs for added flavor and texture.

Note *If freezing for future use, cool the soup, then ladle it into zipper-lock freezer bags or an airtight container, leaving 1 inch (2.5cm) of space at the top. Freeze for up to four months. Thaw the soup in the fridge overnight and heat it on the stovetop, adding a bit of water or broth as needed.*

CHIPOTLE BUTTERNUT SQUASH & PLANTAIN BOWL
WITH SPICY CRANBERRY SAUCE

Rachael: I went to Appalachian State University, which is located in the little mountain town of Boone, North Carolina. We've had several family vacations spent here during my pregnancies, and every time we come, we go to the restaurant Coyote Kitchen because I crave it. They specialize in boats and bowls made up of Caribbean soul food, so we took inspiration from some of our favorite dishes on the menu and created our own bowl. If you ever find yourself in Boone, NC, you now have at least one restaurant to try.

SERVINGS: 9	PREP TIME: 15 MINUTES	TOTAL TIME: 1 HOUR

1 small butternut squash; peeled, seeded, and cubed
2 tablespoons olive oil
1 tablespoon chipotle powder
1 teaspoon smoked paprika
1 teaspoon garlic powder
Salt and pepper, to taste

FOR THE COCONUT RICE
1½ cups jasmine rice
1 (14-ounce/397g) can full-fat coconut milk, well shaken
1¼ cups water
2 tablespoons coconut sugar
1 teaspoon salt
1 teaspoon coconut oil

FOR THE SWEET PLANTAINS
2 tablespoons coconut oil or avocado oil
2 ripe plantains, peeled and sliced into ½-inch-thick (1.25cm) rounds
1 tablespoon coconut sugar
Salt, to taste

FOR THE SAUCE
1 (7-ounce/198g) can chipotle peppers in adobo sauce
1½ cups fresh or frozen cranberries
1 cup water
½ cup pure maple syrup
⅓ cup cane sugar or granulated sugar
Pinch salt

SERVING OPTIONS
Black beans, warmed
Charred corn
Avocado slices
Diced tomato
Cooked shredded chicken

1 **Prepare your rice.** Start by rinsing your rice. Then place rinsed rice, coconut milk, water, coconut sugar, and salt in a medium saucepan. Stir until sugar dissolves, about 1 minute. Place the saucepan over medium heat and bring mixture to a boil. Place a lid on the saucepan, reduce the heat to low, and simmer undisturbed for 11 minutes. Turn off the heat and, keeping the cover on, allow the rice to steam until the rice is tender and the liquid is absorbed, about 10 minutes. Uncover and gently stir in coconut oil. Set aside.

2 Make the chipotle butternut squash while the rice is cooking. Preheat the oven to 400°F (200°C).

3 In a large bowl, toss the cubed butternut squash with olive oil, chipotle powder, smoked paprika, garlic powder, salt, and pepper until evenly coated.

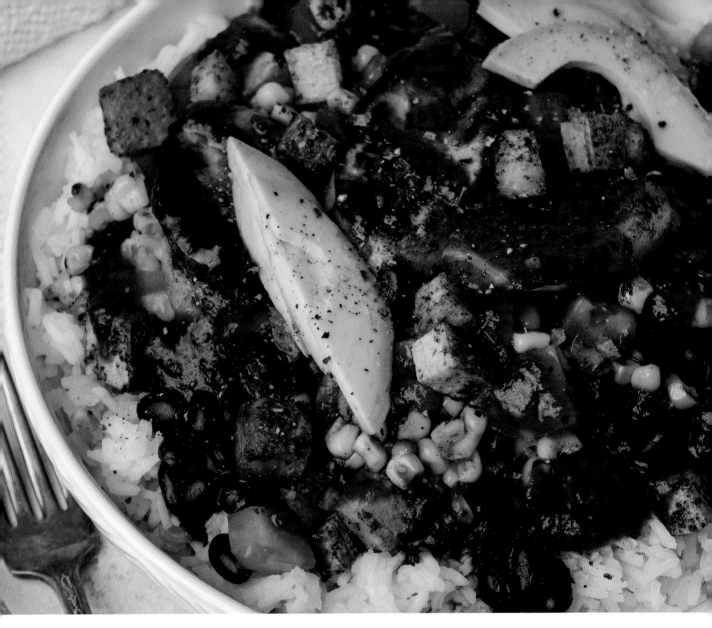

4 Spread the seasoned butternut squash in a single layer onto a large baking sheet lined with parchment paper. Roast for 25 to 30 minutes, until tender and caramelized, flipping halfway through. Remove from the oven and set aside.

5 **Cook the plantains.** Heat coconut oil in a small skillet over medium heat. Add the plantain slices to the skillet and cook for 2 to 3 minutes on each side, until golden brown. Remove the skillet from the heat and sprinkle plantains with coconut sugar.

6 Transfer the cooked plantains to a plate lined with paper towels to drain excess oil. Sprinkle with salt while still warm. Set aside

7 **Make the sauce.** Add the entire can of chipotles in adobo sauce to a blender and blend until smooth.

8 In a medium saucepan over medium heat, add the cranberries, 1 cup water, maple syrup, cane sugar, pinch of salt, and 1½ tablespoons of the blended chipotles. Bring to a simmer and cook for 10 to 15 minutes, until the sauce has reduced and thickened, and the cranberries have popped and broken down.

9 **Create the bowls.** Add about ⅓ cup of rice to each bowl and then layer each bowl evenly with baked chipotle butternut squash and sweet plantains. If desired, add black beans, charred corn, avocado slices, diced tomatoes, and cooked shredded chicken to the bowls. Finish with a drizzle of sauce over the top.

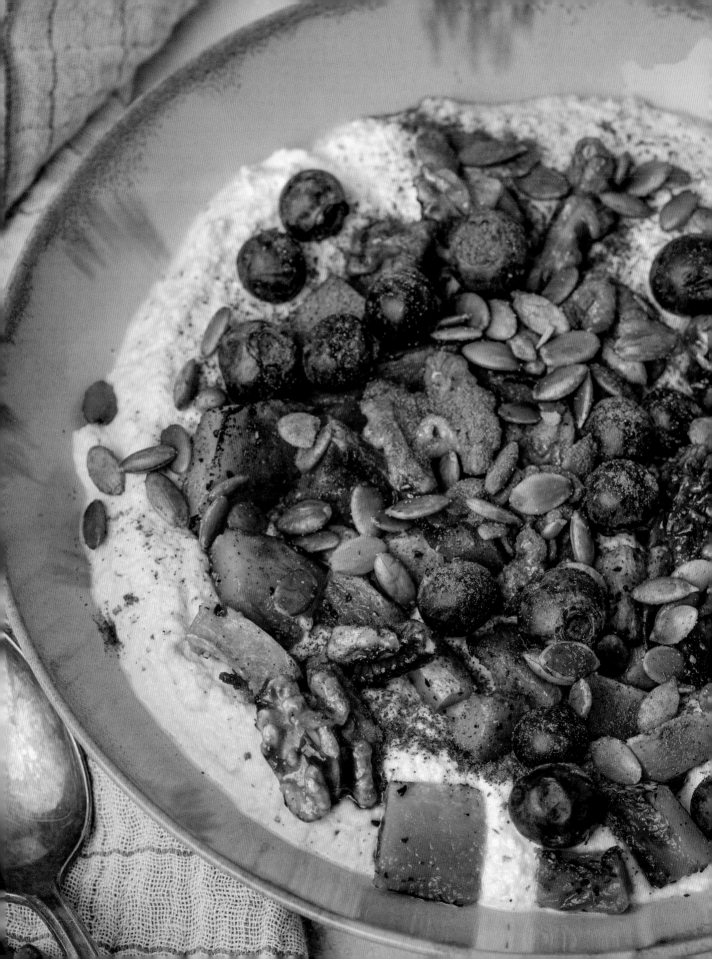

SHEET PAN BUTTERNUT SQUASH & LEMON CASHEW YOGURT

Rachael: One thing I can confidently say during pregnancy, above all else, is that I hated when people told me what to do or how to do something. That's why this dish is completely up to you on when and how you choose to enjoy it. Is it to be had as a dessert? A snack? Prepared for breakfast, lunch, or dinner? To which I answer: it's the dealer's choice. You know your appetite best! If you love a good yogurt bowl, this recipe is its elevated sister that belongs on a restaurant menu. The base is made of a lemon cashew yogurt topped with roasted butternut squash, walnuts, and a few (suggested) toppings.

SERVINGS: 2–4	PREP TIME: 10 MINUTES	TOTAL TIME: 40 MINUTES

1 medium butternut squash; peeled, seeded, and cut into ½-inch (1.25cm) cubes
1 tablespoons olive oil
3 tablespoons maple syrup, divided
1½ teaspoons ground nutmeg
1½ teaspoons ground cinnamon
Salt and pepper, to taste
1 cup walnuts

FOR THE LEMON CASHEW YOGURT
½ cup raw cashews, soaked in water for at least 4 hours or overnight
¼ cup water
2 tablespoons lemon juice
1 tablespoon chopped fresh parsley
1 tablespoon chopped fresh cilantro
Salt and pepper, to taste

SERVING OPTIONS
1 cup roasted pumpkin seeds
½ cup fresh blueberries
Pinch of ground cinnamon

1 Preheat the oven to 400°F (200°C).

2 Place the cubed butternut squash on a large baking sheet lined with parchment paper.

3 Drizzle with olive oil and 2 tablespoons maple syrup and then season with nutmeg, cinnamon, salt, and pepper, tossing to coat evenly.

4 Roast for 35 to 40 minutes, until the squash is tender and lightly browned, stirring halfway through.

5 While the squash roasts, prepare the walnuts by placing a skillet over medium heat. Add the walnuts, remaining 1 tablespoon maple syrup, and a pinch of salt. Cook, stirring frequently, until syrup is caramelized and nuts are toasted, about 3 minutes. Let cool and set aside.

6 **Prepare the lemon cashew yogurt.** Drain the soaked cashews and rinse them thoroughly.

7 In a blender, combine the soaked cashews, water, lemon juice, parsley, and cilantro. Blend until smooth and creamy. Add more water if needed to reach your desired consistency. Season with salt and pepper to taste.

8 To serve, spoon the lemon cashew yogurt onto a serving platter and add the butternut squash and walnuts on top of the yogurt. Garnish with the roasted pumpkin seeds, fresh blueberries, and an additional pinch of cinnamon, if desired.

BUTTERNUT SQUASH RISOTTO

Tom: Making risotto demands continuous attention and care, much like what shortly awaits you with a new little one. As I write, we have one child and another on the way. I expect it will differ from our first experience, but those initial three weeks left lifelong memories and emotions. There are also significant time gaps in my memories, likely due to sleep deprivation! So, let's enjoy this elegant meal and embrace the challenges and joys that are around the corner.

SERVINGS: 3–4	PREP TIME: 10 MINUTES	TOTAL TIME: 45 MINUTES

1 small butternut squash; peeled, seeded, and diced into small cubes
4 tablespoons olive oil, divided
Salt and pepper, to taste
4 cups vegetable broth or chicken broth
1 tablespoon unsalted butter
1 small white onion, finely chopped
2 garlic cloves, minced
1½ cups Arborio rice
½ cup dry white wine
½ cup grated Parmesan or ¼ cup nutritional yeast if dairy-free
Fried sage

1 Preheat the oven to 400°F (200°C).

2 Place the diced butternut squash on a baking sheet lined with parchment paper. Drizzle with 2 tablespoons of olive oil and season with salt and pepper. Toss to coat evenly.

3 Roast for 25 to 30 minutes, until the squash is tender and caramelized, flipping halfway through, then remove from the oven and set aside. While the squash is roasting proceed with starting the risotto.

4 In a medium saucepan, heat the vegetable broth over medium heat. Once heated, reduce the heat to low to keep it warm.

5 In a large skillet or Dutch oven, heat the remaining 2 tablespoons of olive oil and the butter over medium heat.

6 Add the onion and garlic to the skillet. Cook until the onion is soft and translucent, about 3 to 4 minutes.

7 Add the Arborio rice to the skillet and cook, stirring constantly, for 1 to 2 minutes until the rice is well coated with oil and slightly toasted.

8 Pour in the white wine and cook, stirring, until the wine has evaporated and the alcohol has cooked off, another 1 to 2 minutes.

9 Begin adding the warm broth to the skillet, one ladleful at a time, stirring frequently and allowing the liquid to absorb before adding another ladleful. Continue this process until the rice is cooked through and creamy, about 20 to 25 minutes.

10 Once the risotto is almost done, fold in the roasted butternut squash cubes until evenly distributed, reserving ¼ cup of cooked butternut squash for garnish. Cook for an additional 2 to 3 minutes to heat through.

11 Remove the skillet from heat and stir in the grated Parmesan. Season with additional salt and pepper, to taste.

12 Serve the risotto hot, garnished with the reserved ¼ cup butternut squash, as well as fried sage and additional Parmesan, if desired.

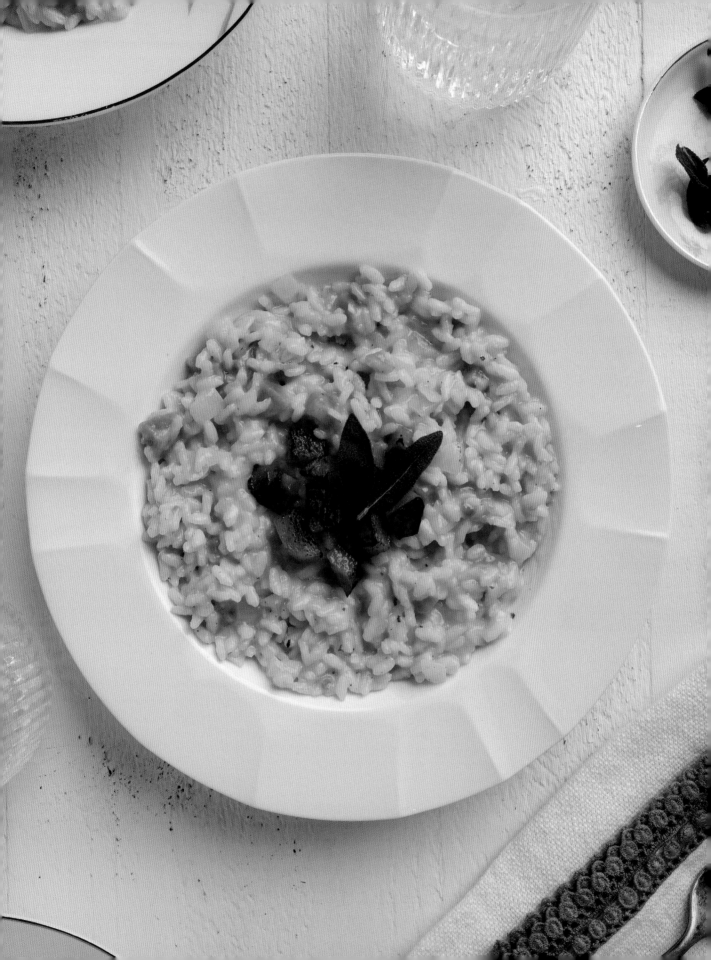

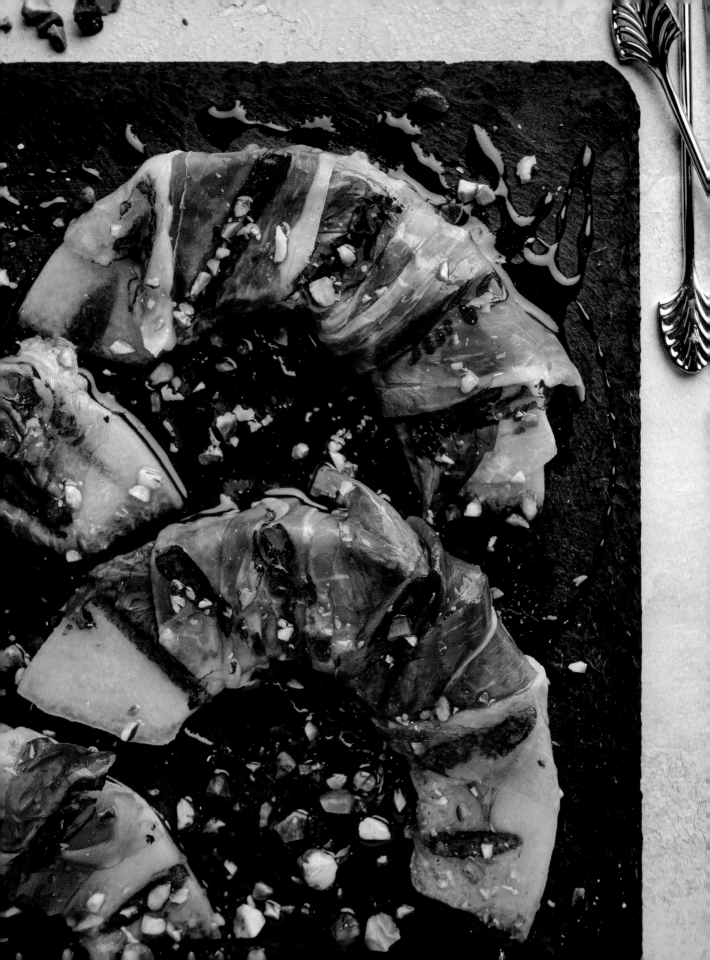

GRILLED PROSCIUTTO-WRAPPED CANTALOUPE

WITH HONEY

Tom: I love when you can take five ingredients and with simple steps make an effortless appetizer that is sophisticated and sure to impress. Each bite starts with the salty prosciutto covering a juicy wedge of cantaloupe, paired with fresh basil, and finished with the subtle smoke of the grill. The dish is enhanced with a drizzle of sweet honey and the crunch of chopped pistachios. Ideal for entertaining or for a quick snack.

SERVINGS: 4–6	PREP TIME: 15 MINUTES	TOTAL TIME: 25 MINUTES

6–8 slices prosciutto, cut in half lengthwise

1 small ripe cantaloupe; peeled, seeded, and cut into ½-inch-thick (1.25cm) wedges

12–16 fresh basil leaves

1–2 tablespoons raw honey

½ cup roughly chopped pistachios, optional

Toothpicks or small skewers

1 Preheat the grill to 450°F (230°C) or place a large grill pan over medium-high heat.

2 Lay a strip of prosciutto flat. Place a wedge of cantaloupe at one end of the prosciutto slice. Place a basil leaf on the cantaloupe, then roll the prosciutto around the cantaloupe wedge securing the basil tightly. Repeat with the remaining prosciutto slices, cantaloupe wedges, and basil leaves.

3 Grill the prosciutto-wrapped cantaloupe for 3 minutes per side.

4 Arrange the prosciutto-wrapped cantaloupe on a serving platter. Drizzle the raw honey over the top of the wrapped cantaloupe. You can adjust the amount of honey based on your preference for sweetness.

5 If desired, garnish with chopped pistachios.

6 Insert toothpicks into each prosciutto-wrapped cantaloupe wedge for easy serving. Serve immediately as an appetizer or snack.

YOGURT TOAST
WITH CANTALOUPE RIBBONS

Rachael: There are weeks of pregnancy that fly by and some that stand out amongst the rest. During my first pregnancy, this week stands out to me. It wasn't anything significant, like finding out the baby's sex or seeing the baby during an anatomy scan. Tom was just having a creative week in the kitchen. Our love felt strong. The realization that it wasn't going to be just us anymore was settling in. I was on a yogurt toast kick at the time, so Tom used his mandoline to make these cantaloupe ribbons and that ended up being the perfect pairing to a sweet and memorable week.

SERVINGS: 2	PREP TIME: 10 MINUTES	TOTAL TIME: 3 HOURS 20 MINUTES

½ cup unsweetened cashew yogurt or Greek yogurt

½ tablespoon raw honey

Dash of vanilla extract

2 bacon slices

½ small ripe cantaloupe, peel and seeds removed

½ tablespoon coconut oil

2 slices gluten-free bread of choice

4 strawberries, thinly sliced

SERVING OPTIONS

Raw honey

Fresh mint leaves

Pinch of ground cinnamon

1 In a bowl, mix the yogurt, honey and vanilla extract. Cover and place in the fridge to chill.

2 Place a small skillet over medium high heat and cook your bacon until crispy. Remove bacon to a paper towel to cool and then break it into pieces.

3 Using a vegetable peeler, carefully peel thin ribbons of cantaloupe from the flesh. Continue peeling until you have enough ribbons to cover both slices of toast. Set aside.

4 Place a small pan over medium heat. Add the coconut oil and toast your bread for 2 to 3 minutes per side until golden brown. Remove toast from the pan.

5 Spread a generous layer of the yogurt mix on each slice of toasted bread. Layer the yogurt with strawberry slices, then cantaloupe ribbons, and top with bacon pieces.

6 If desired, drizzle additional raw honey over the cantaloupe ribbons for added sweetness, and sprinkle chopped fresh mint leaves and a pinch of cinnamon over the yogurt and cantaloupe for a pop of color and extra flavor.

7 Enjoy whole or slice the toast in half before serving.

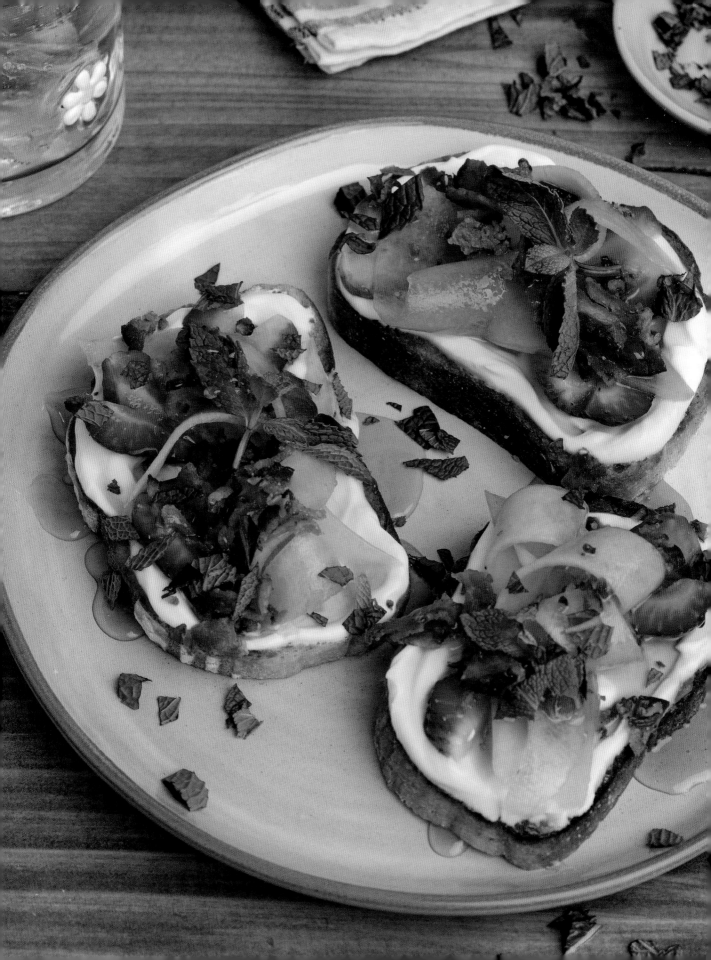

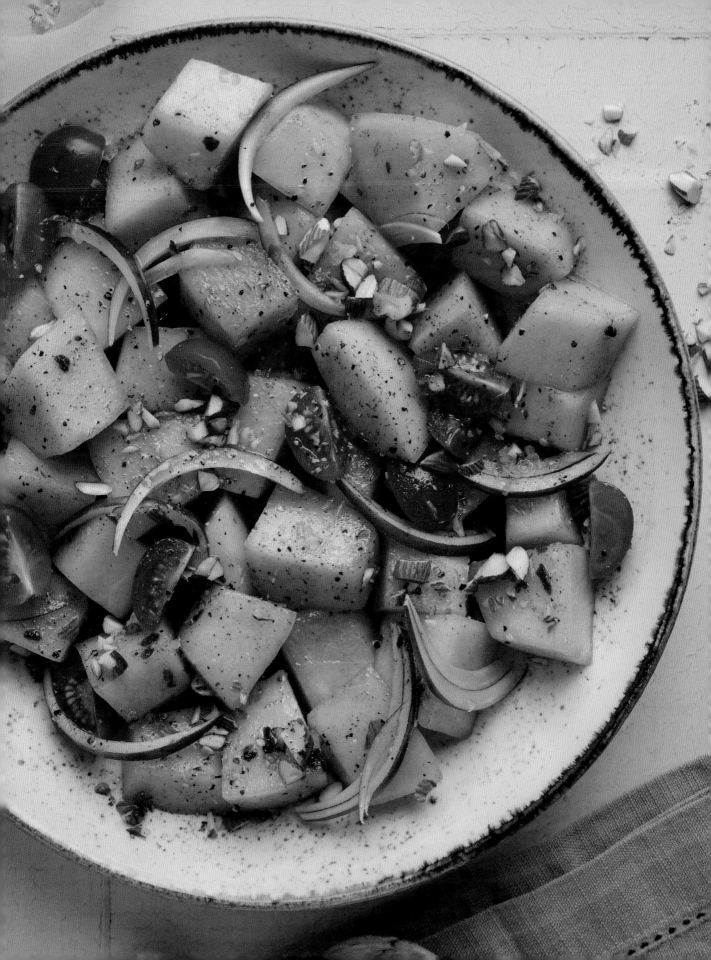

— week 36 —

CANTALOUPE & HERB SALAD
WITH CHILI-LIME VINAIGRETTE

Tom: This week, your baby's immune system is gearing up for life outside of your womb, so we made a salad that contains a variety of fresh herbs, which are rich sources of vitamins A, C, and K, as well as minerals like iron and calcium that are vital for maintaining overall health and supporting the baby's immune system.

SERVINGS: 2–3	PREP TIME: 15 MINUTES	TOTAL TIME: 15 MINUTES

1 small ripe cantaloupe; peeled, seeded, and cubed
¼ cup toasted almond pieces
6-8 cherry tomatoes, quartered
¼ medium red onion, thinly sliced

FOR THE DRESSING
2 tablespoons olive oil
1 tablespoon honey
1 tablespoon lime juice
½ teaspoon red pepper flakes
¼ teaspoon ground cumin
½ teaspoon paprika
½ teaspoon onion powder
½ teaspoon garlic powder
Salt and pepper, to taste

SERVING OPTIONS
2 cups mixed salad greens, such as arugula, spinach, or mixed baby greens
Fresh basil leaves
Fresh mint leaves
Chopped fresh cilantro

1 In a large salad bowl, combine the cantaloupe cubes, toasted almonds, cherry tomatoes, and red onion.

2 **Prepare the dressing.** In a small bowl, whisk together all the dressing ingredients until well combined. Season with salt and pepper to taste.

3 Drizzle the dressing over the salad ingredients in the bowl. Toss gently until everything is evenly coated with the dressing.

4 If desired, add salad greens, basil, mint, and cilantro to taste.

5 Divide onto individual serving plates or bowls and serve immediately.

RHUBARB-GLAZED CHICKEN WINGS

Rachael: I don't know how we've made it this far into the book without a wing recipe. For those of you pregnant during the football season, which covers fall and winter in the United States, I can't picture a better Sunday meal. Whether you watch sports or not, most of us can get behind the food spread on game day. If you are pregnant during summer, this is a delicious choice to bring to that backyard barbecue. If you are pregnant during spring, lucky you! Rhubarb is in season, and you get to experience the freshest tart-and-tangy version of this recipe.

SERVINGS: 4	**PREP TIME:** 10 MINUTES	**TOTAL TIME:** 55 MINUTES

2 pounds (907g) chicken wings, split at the joints, tips removed
1 cup diced fresh rhubarb
¼ cup honey or maple syrup
2 tablespoons apple cider vinegar
1 tablespoon olive oil
2 garlic cloves, minced
1 teaspoon grated fresh ginger
Salt and pepper

SERVING OPTIONS
Chopped green onions
Toasted sesame seeds

1 Preheat the oven or air fryer to 400°F (200°C) and line a baking sheet with parchment paper.

2 In a small saucepan, combine the rhubarb, honey, apple cider vinegar, olive oil, garlic, ginger, and a pinch of salt and pepper. Cook over medium heat, stirring occasionally, until the rhubarb breaks down and the mixture thickens slightly, about 10 to 15 minutes. Remove from heat and set aside.

3 Pat the chicken wings dry with paper towels and season with salt and pepper to preference. Place the wings on the prepared baking sheet in a single layer. Place in the preheated oven and bake for 20 minutes. Remove from the oven, leaving the oven on.

4 Using a pastry brush or spoon, generously brush the rhubarb glaze over the chicken wings, coating them evenly, and then flip the wings and glaze the other side.

5 Return the baking sheet to the oven and bake for 5 to 10 additional minutes, until the chicken wings are cooked through to an internal temperature of 165°F (74°C). (See note.)

6 Once the chicken wings are cooked through, remove them from the oven or air fryer and garnish with chopped green onions and sesame seeds, if desired. Allow them to cool slightly before serving.

Note *Alternatively, you can air-fry the wings for 8 minutes on each side instead of placing them back in the oven.*

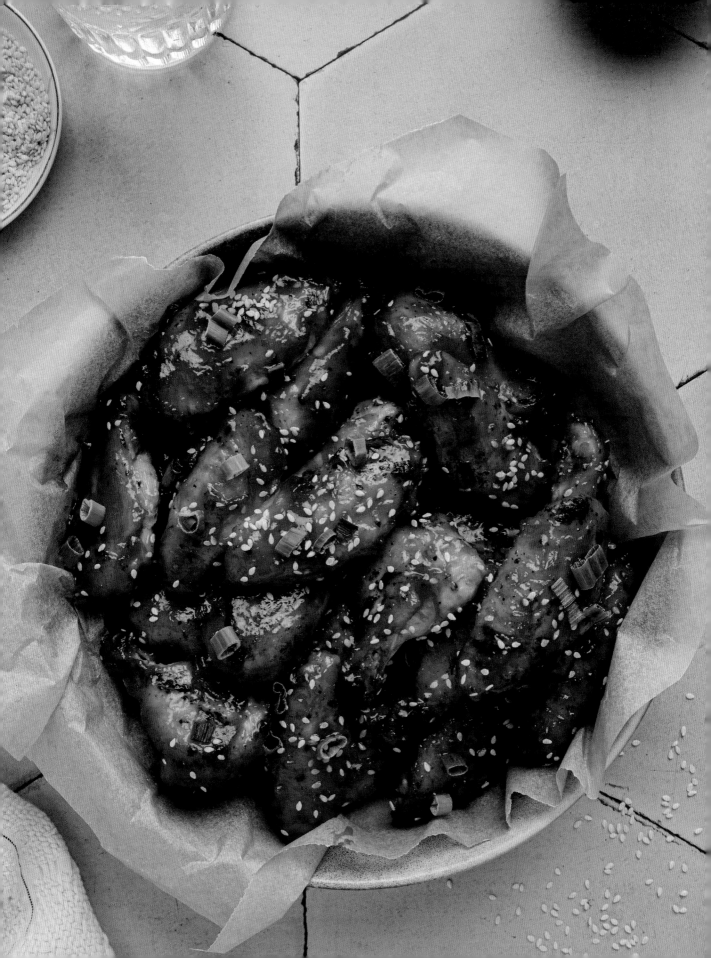

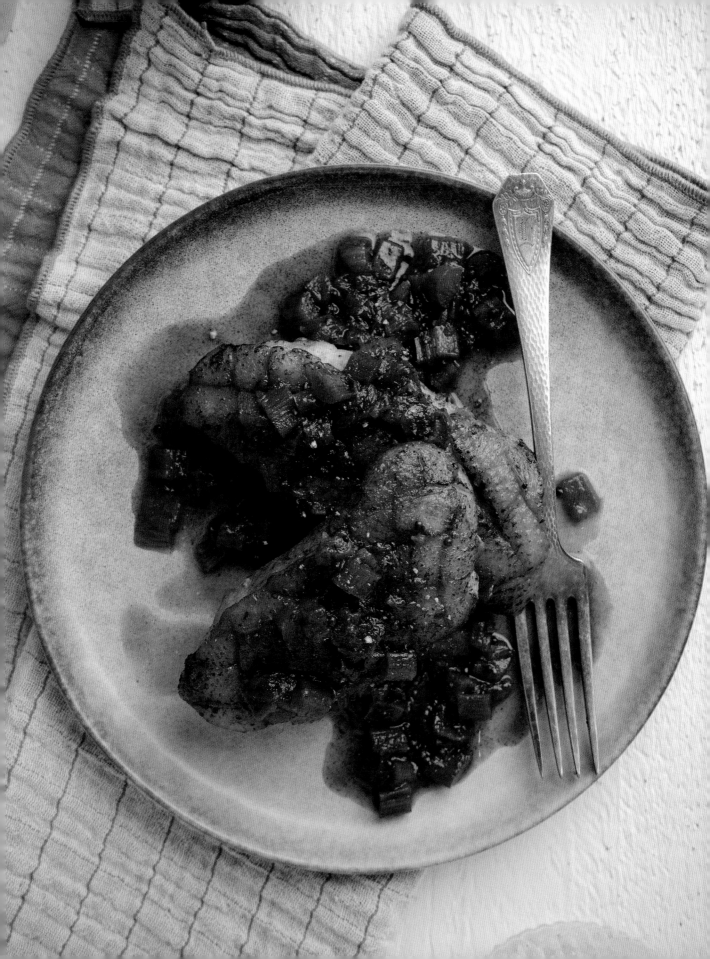

CRISPY DUCK BREAST

WITH RHUBARB CHUTNEY

Tom: I recently ran an Instagram poll and discovered that about 85% of poll takers haven't cooked duck at home yet. If you're among the majority who haven't tried it, get excited! Cooking duck might seem daunting, but it's actually quite straightforward and gives you the feeling of being a Michelin star chef right in your own kitchen. This recipe beautifully pairs the rich, savory flavors of crispy duck breast with a sweet and slightly tangy rhubarb chutney. It's designed to be both impressive and accessible, offering a gourmet touch without requiring advanced skills. Perfect for a special date night to celebrate your growing family.

SERVINGS: 2	PREP TIME: 10 MINUTES	TOTAL TIME: 55 MINUTES

2 duck breasts, 6-8 ounces (179-227g) each
Salt and pepper, to taste

FOR THE CHUTNEY
2 cups diced fresh rhubarb
½ cup diced red onion
¼ cup maple syrup
¼ cup apple cider vinegar
2 tablespoons grated fresh ginger
1 teaspoon mustard seeds
½ teaspoon ground cinnamon
¼ teaspoon ground allspice
Salt and pepper, to taste

1 **Prepare the chutney.** In a medium saucepan, combine all the chutney ingredients.

2 Bring the mixture to a simmer over medium heat, then reduce the heat to low and let it cook, stirring occasionally, until the rhubarb is soft and the mixture has reduced and thickened slightly, about 20 to 25 minutes. Remove from heat and set aside.

3 **Prepare the duck breasts.** Score the skin of the duck breasts with a sharp knife in a ½-inch (1.25cm) crosshatch pattern, being careful not to cut into the meat. This helps the fat render during cooking.

4 Season both sides of the duck breasts generously with salt and pepper.

5 Place the duck breasts skin side down in a large cold skillet and place over medium high heat. Once the skillet is hot, cook for 5 to 7 minutes or until the skin is crispy and golden brown.

6 Flip the duck breasts and continue to cook for another 7 to 10 minutes or until an internal temperature of 165°F (74°C) is reached.

7 Remove the duck breasts from the skillet and let them rest for at least 5 minutes before slicing.

8 Slice the duck breasts and serve with a generous spoonful of rhubarb chutney on top. Our favorite side dishes for this recipe include roasted vegetables or mashed sweet potatoes.

RHUBARB, APPLE & ALMOND COBBLER

Rachael: This could be the last dessert you make before the baby is delivered. Isn't it crazy to think we are at that point? Remember when you were just making blueberry skillet pancakes, and now we're here? Soak in all the sweetness of this week with this rhubarb, apple, and almond cobbler. It's a little nutty, sweet, and tart all wrapped into one warm bite ... a heaping spoonful of ice cream on top never hurt anyone either.

SERVINGS: 8	PREP TIME: 15 MINUTES	TOTAL TIME: 50 MINUTES

1 teaspoon coconut oil or butter
3 cups diced fresh rhubarb
2 cups diced baking apples, such as Granny Smith or Honeycrisp
¼ cup honey or maple syrup
1 tablespoon lemon juice
1 teaspoon ground cinnamon
½ teaspoon ground ginger
¼ teaspoon ground nutmeg
2 tablespoons arrowroot powder or cornstarch

FOR THE ALMOND TOPPING
1 cup almond flour
½ cup gluten-free rolled oats
¼ cup chopped almonds
¼ cup honey or maple syrup
¼ cup coconut oil or butter, melted
1 teaspoon vanilla extract
½ teaspoon ground cinnamon
Pinch of salt

SERVING OPTIONS
Vanilla ice cream or dairy-free ice cream
Coconut whipped cream

1 Preheat the oven to 350°F (180°C). Grease a 9x9-inch (23x23cm) baking dish with coconut oil.

2 Prepare the filling. In a large mixing bowl, combine rhubarb, apples, honey, lemon juice, cinnamon, ginger, nutmeg, and arrowroot powder. Toss until the fruit is evenly coated.

3 Transfer the rhubarb-apple mixture to the prepared baking dish, spreading it out evenly.

4 **Prepare the almond topping.** In another medium mixing bowl, combine almond flour, oats, almonds, honey, coconut oil, vanilla extract, cinnamon, and salt. Mix until well combined and crumbly.

5 Sprinkle the almond topping evenly over the rhubarb-apple mixture in the baking dish.

6 Transfer the baking dish to the preheated oven and bake for 30 to 35 minutes, until the filling is bubbling and the cobbler topping is golden brown and crisp.

7 Remove the cobbler from the oven and let it cool for a few minutes before serving. Serve warm, with a scoop of vanilla ice cream and coconut whipped cream on top, if desired.

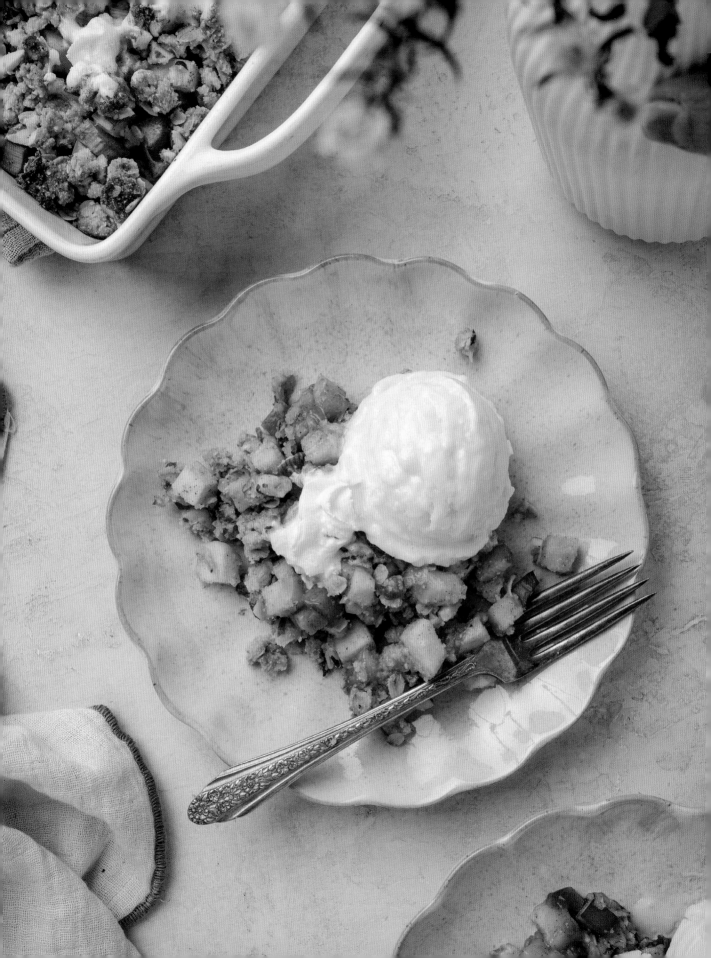

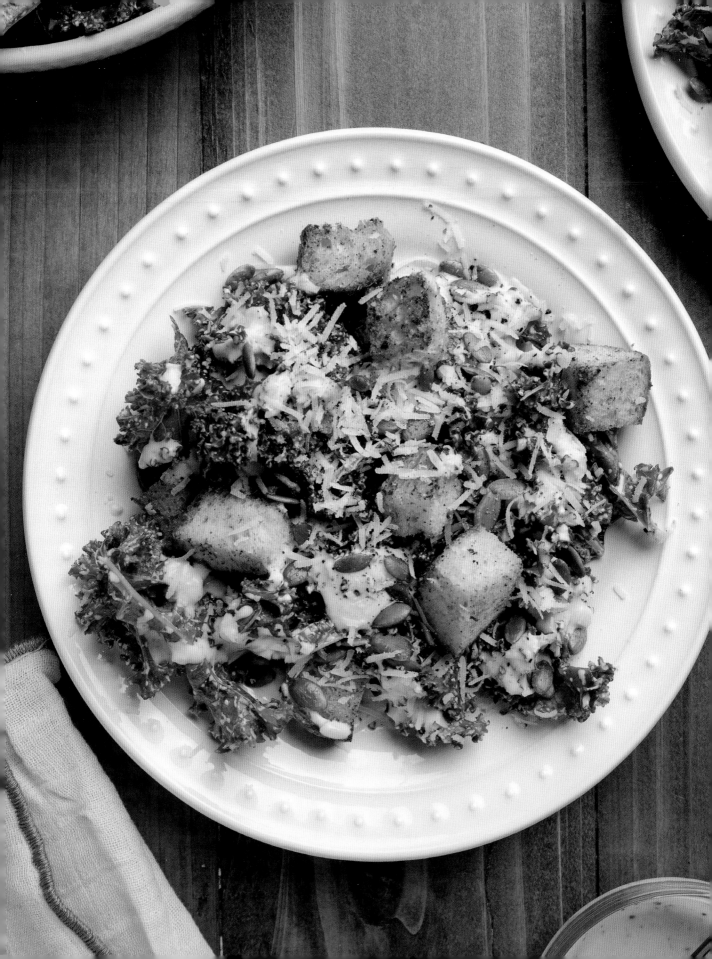

KALE CAESAR SALAD

Tom: This is a fair warning, once you make this Caesar dressing, you will have a very hard time using store-bought dressing again. This meal is simple and healthy with a fresh and crunchy bite to it. We typically make four times the amount of dressing and use it in several recipes throughout the week.

SERVINGS: 2	PREP TIME: 15 MINUTES	TOTAL TIME: 15 MINUTES

1 bunch of kale, stems removed and leaves torn into bite-size pieces

½ cup mayonnaise

4 tablespoons extra-virgin olive oil, divided

2 tablespoons lemon juice

1 tablespoon Dijon mustard

1 garlic clove, minced

1 anchovy fillet, mashed, or 1 teaspoon anchovy paste, optional

½ teaspoon salt

1½ teaspoons freshly cracked black pepper

¼ cup grated Parmesan or nutritional yeast for a dairy-free option

SERVING OPTIONS
Roasted pumpkin seeds (pepitas)

Grilled chicken breast, sliced

Croutons

Cherry tomato halves

1 Place the torn kale leaves in a large salad bowl with 2 tablespoons olive oil. Massage the kale with your hands for a few minutes until it is well coated and becomes tender and slightly wilted. Move to the refrigerator.

2 In a small bowl, whisk together the mayonnaise, remaining 2 tablespoons olive oil, lemon juice, Dijon mustard, minced garlic, mashed anchovy fillet (if using), salt, and black pepper until well combined. Adjust the salt and pepper to taste.

3 Remove the massaged kale from the refrigerator. Pour the dressing over the kale and toss until the kale leaves are evenly coated.

4 Sprinkle the grated Parmesan over the dressed kale. If desired, add roasted pumpkin seeds, slices of grilled chicken breast, croutons, or cherry tomato halves.

5 Divide the salad into individual bowls and serve immediately.

Note *Store any extra dressing in an airtight container in the refrigerator for up to a week. Shake before using. If preferred, avocado oil mayonnaise works well in this recipe.*

BAKED KALE FRITTATA

Rachael: This kale frittata has not only an excellent source of vitamins and nutrients to support the baby while still in the womb, but it's an amazing postpartum meal to have on hand too. During postpartum, you want to focus on foods containing nutrients that support energy and healing, but are also convenient. This is a dish you can keep stored in the fridge to heat up for breakfast. You're gonna need to sustain as much energy as possible in the weeks and months coming off pregnancy, so make choices that are going to best serve you and your body's well-being.

SERVINGS: 4–6	PREP TIME: 10 MINUTES	TOTAL TIME: 40 MINUTES

1 tablespoon olive oil
½ yellow onion, thinly sliced
1 garlic clove, minced
2 cups chopped kale leaves
Salt and pepper, to taste
8 large eggs
¼ cup unsweetened almond milk or any milk of your choice

OPTIONAL ADD-INS
Diced bell pepper
Sliced mushrooms
Cherry tomatoes halves

Note *Store leftover frittata wedges in an airtight container in the fridge for up to 4 days.*

1 Preheat the oven to 350°F (180°C).

2 In a large ovenproof skillet, heat the olive oil over medium heat. Add the onion and garlic, and sauté until softened and fragrant, about 3 to 4 minutes.

3 Add the chopped kale to the skillet and continue to cook until the kale wilts, about 3 to 4 minutes. Season with salt and pepper to taste. If you are including any optional add-ins, put them in the skillet now and sauté until they're tender.

4 In a large mixing bowl, whisk together the eggs and almond milk until well combined. Season with additional salt and pepper.

5 Pour the whisked eggs over the sautéed kale and onions in the skillet. Use a spatula to gently distribute the kale and onions evenly throughout the egg mixture.

6 Quickly transfer the skillet to the preheated oven and bake for 15 to 20 minutes, until the frittata is set in the center and the edges are lightly golden brown.

7 Once cooked through, remove the frittata from the oven and let it cool for a few minutes. Slice into wedges and serve warm. This kale frittata is delicious served on its own or paired with a side salad for a complete meal.

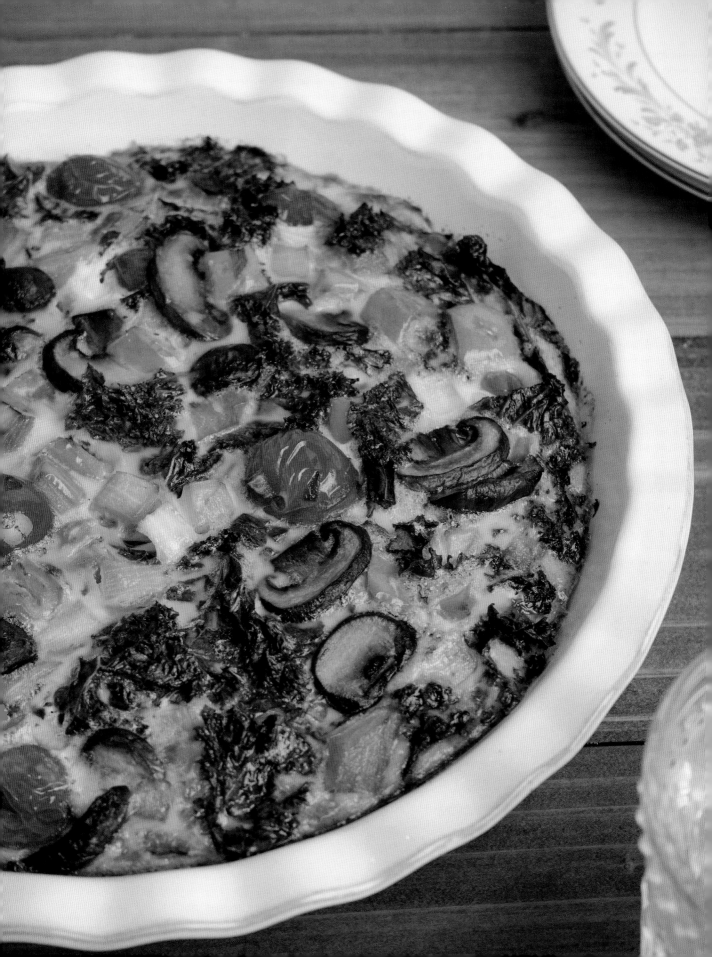

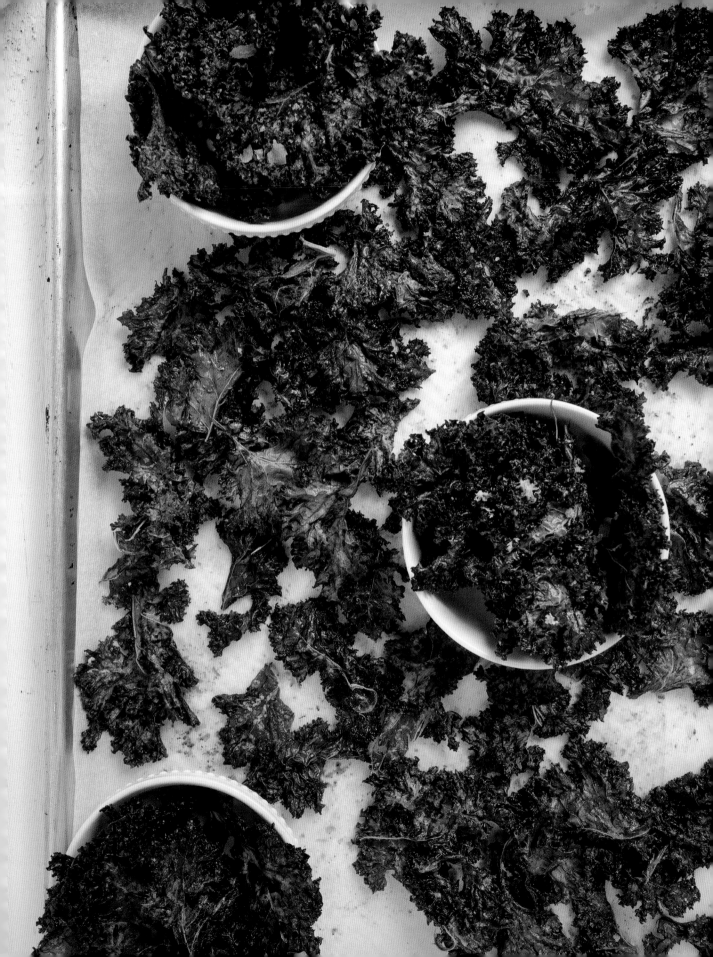

KALE CHIPS, FOUR WAYS

Rachael: A top prenatal superfood packed with nutrients, kale is the perfect ingredient to sneak into your pregnancy diet ... so let's make some kale chips! I started making kale chips in college and fell in love with them. I love eating them alone as a snack, but I also love using them to top protein bowls for some added crunch and nutrients.

SERVINGS: 4	PREP TIME: 5 MINUTES	TOTAL TIME: 25 MINUTES

1 bunch of kale, stems removed and torn into bite-size pieces
2 tablespoons olive oil

FOR CLASSIC SEA SALT AND VINEGAR KALE CHIPS
2 tablespoons apple cider vinegar
Salt, to taste

FOR "CHEESY" GARLIC KALE CHIPS
2 tablespoons nutritional yeast
1 teaspoon garlic powder
Salt, to taste

FOR SPICY PAPRIKA KALE CHIPS
1 teaspoon smoked paprika
½ teaspoon chili powder
Salt, to taste

FOR TANGY LEMON-PEPPER KALE CHIPS
Zest of 1 lemon
½ teaspoon black pepper
Salt, to taste

1 Preheat the oven to 300°F (150°C) and line a large baking sheet with parchment paper.

2 In a large mixing bowl, toss the torn kale pieces with olive oil until evenly coated. Massage the kale gently with your hands to ensure the oil is well distributed.

3 **FOR CLASSIC SEA SALT AND VINEGAR KALE CHIPS**
Drizzle the apple cider vinegar over the kale, then sprinkle with salt to taste.
FOR CHEESY GARLIC KALE CHIPS
Sprinkle the nutritional yeast and garlic powder over the kale, tossing to coat evenly, then add salt to taste.
FOR SPICY PAPRIKA KALE CHIPS
Sprinkle the smoked paprika and chili powder over the kale, tossing to coat evenly, then add salt to taste.
FOR TANGY LEMON-PEPPER KALE CHIPS
Sprinkle the lemon zest and black pepper over the kale, tossing to coat evenly, then add salt to taste.

4 Spread the seasoned kale pieces in a single layer on the prepared baking sheet, making sure they're not overlapping.

5 Bake for 15 to 20 minutes, until the kale chips are crispy and slightly golden brown, checking frequently to prevent burning.

6 Remove the kale chips from the oven and let them cool on the baking sheet for a few minutes before serving.

— week 39 —

SAVORY PUMPKIN PASTA SAUCE

Rachael: At this point, the baby is just waiting for the right time to make their appearance into the world, and if you make this pumpkin pasta sauce, there's a chance they may never want to leave. On a serious note, there is a lot of anxiety and excitement that you may be feeling. I was so scared for the baby to make its arrival because this chapter of my life would officially close and a new one would start. I remember seeing and hearing everyone else who was at this stage of pregnancy ready to be done with pregnancy, and I felt anything but. So if you are a little nervous, just know you are not alone, but you do only have a week of recipes left to go.

SERVINGS: 4–5	**PREP TIME:** 5 MINUTES	**TOTAL TIME:** 25 MINUTES

1 tablespoon olive oil
1 small white onion, finely chopped
2 garlic cloves, minced
1 cup pumpkin purée
1 cup low-sodium vegetable broth or
 chicken broth
½ cup canned coconut milk
1 tablespoon chopped fresh sage or
 1 teaspoon dried sage
Salt and pepper, to taste
¼ teaspoon ground nutmeg, optional
¼ teaspoon ground cinnamon,
 optional
½ teaspoon red pepper flakes, optional

SERVING OPTIONS
Gluten-free pasta of choice, penne or
 gnocchi preferred
Freshly grated Parmesan
Fresh parsley or basil, chopped
Fried sage
Pinch of red pepper flakes

1 In a large skillet over medium heat, add the olive oil. Once hot, add the onion and cook until soft and translucent, about 5 minutes. Add the garlic and cook for another minute, until fragrant.

2 Add the pumpkin purée, broth, and coconut milk to the skillet. Stir well to combine everything thoroughly.

3 Stir in the sage, as well as salt and pepper to taste. Add the nutmeg, cinnamon, and red pepper flakes, if using. Let the sauce simmer for about 10 minutes on low heat, allowing the flavors to meld together. Taste and adjust the seasonings as needed.

4 Serve the sauce over your choice of gluten-free pasta. Grate some Parmesan over the top and finish with a sprinkle of fresh parsley, fried sage, and additional red pepper flakes, if desired.

Note For a heartier sauce, consider adding ground turkey, ground chicken, or Italian sausage to the sauce. Cook it with the onion in step 1, breaking it up with a spoon as it cooks and then draining it, before adding the other ingredients.

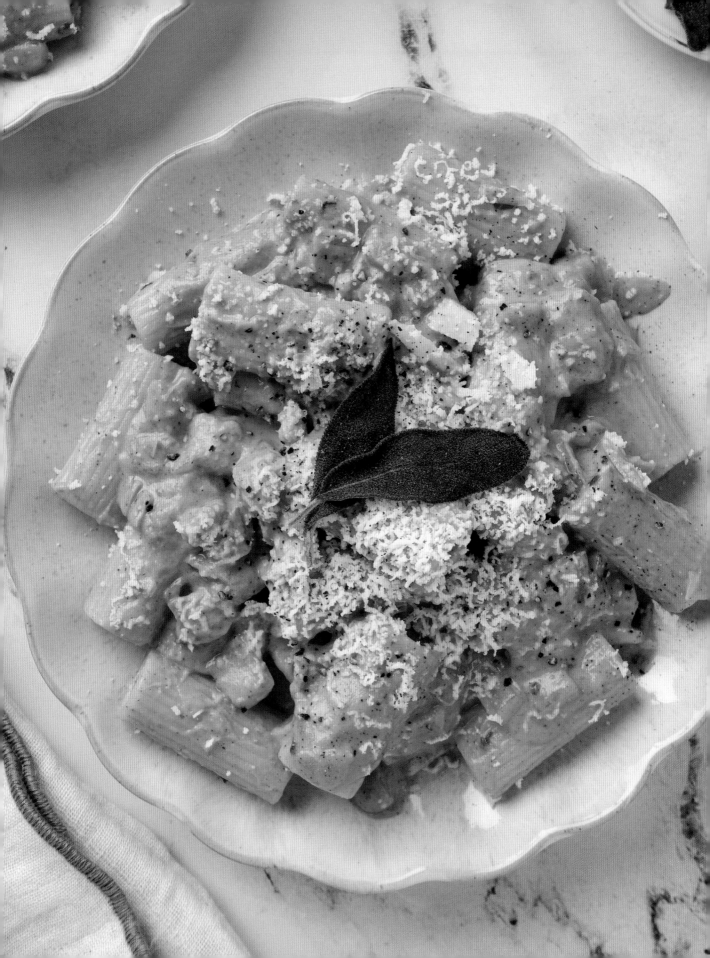

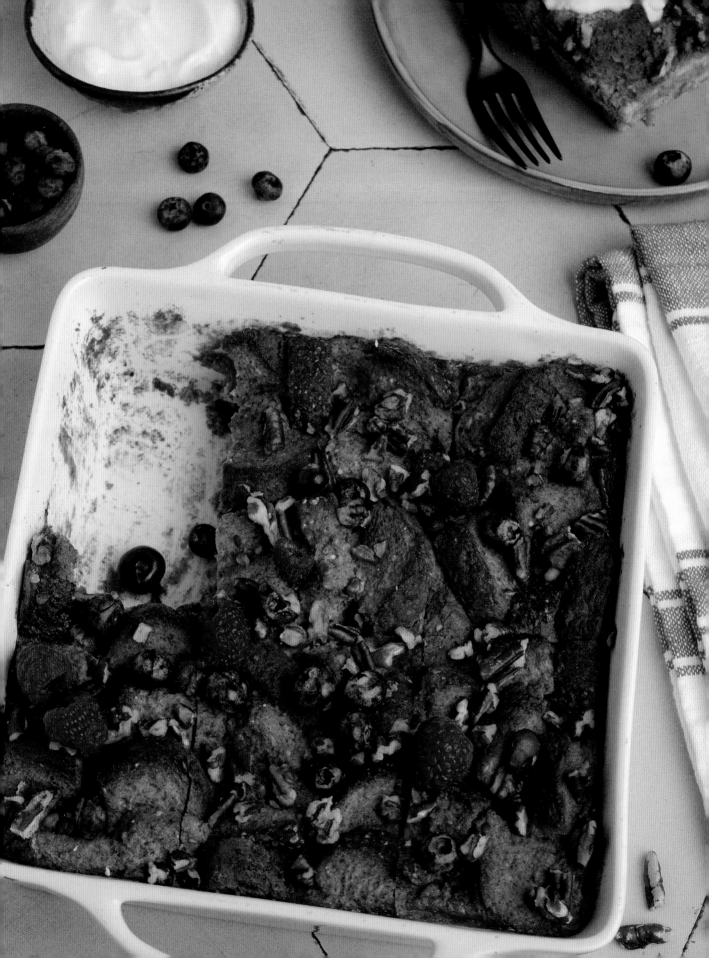

— week 39 —

PUMPKIN FRENCH TOAST CASSEROLE

Rachael: How does it feel to be considered full term? At this point, you might be trying to curb walk that baby out or you might just be so uncomfortable that movement is difficult these days. I know cooking might be the last thing on your mind, so we are going to simplify breakfast this week with a pumpkin french toast casserole. It's as simple as mixing together all of the ingredients in a bowl and then pouring it into a casserole dish. After you make it once, you won't have to worry about breakfast for most of the week, and we want this week to run as smoothly as possible for you!

SERVINGS: 6–8	**PREP TIME**: 25 MINUTES	**TOTAL TIME**: 1 HOUR 20 MINUTES

1 teaspoon olive oil or coconut oil

1 cup canned pumpkin purée

2 cups unsweetened almond milk or any milk of choice

4 large eggs

¼ cup pure maple syrup or honey

1 teaspoon vanilla extract

1 teaspoon ground cinnamon

½ teaspoon ground nutmeg

¼ teaspoon ground ginger

½ teaspoon salt

1 loaf gluten-free bread, cut into 1-inch (2.5cm) cubes, whole-grain preferred

½ cup chopped pecans or walnuts, optional

SERVING OPTIONS

Maple syrup or honey

Greek yogurt or dairy-free yogurt

Fresh berries

Nuts

1 Preheat the oven to 350°F (180°C). Grease a 9x13-inch (23x33cm) baking dish with a teaspoon of olive oil.

2 In a large bowl, whisk together the pumpkin purée, almond milk, eggs, maple syrup, vanilla extract, cinnamon, nutmeg, ginger, and salt until well combined. Fold in your bread cubes, coating thoroughly, and then allow the mixture to soak into the bread for about 20 minutes.

3 Pour the pumpkin and bread cube mixture into your baking dish.

4 Sprinkle the top of the casserole with chopped pecans, if using.

5 Place the casserole in the oven and bake for 45 to 55 minutes, until the top is golden brown and the center is set.

6 Allow the casserole to cool slightly before serving. Serve warm with a drizzle of maple syrup, a dollop of Greek yogurt, and fresh berries or nuts on top, if desired.

Note *Ensure pumpkin purée, not pumpkin-pie filling, is used for this recipe.*

— week 39 —

PUMPKIN OATMEAL

Rachael: Remember during the grape week, when we talked about oats and their importance for postpartum and breastfeeding? Well, we have another oat recipe here, and this is not the instant oatmeal with boiled water I used to eat for breakfast as a kid. It starts with a velvety pumpkin purée; chia seeds for added texture; a blend of cinnamon, nutmeg, and ginger; and a hint of sweetness from maple syrup. It's a cozy bowl of goodness that tastes like fall is on the way.

SERVINGS: 2	PREP TIME: 5 MINUTES	TOTAL TIME: 15 MINUTES

½ cup gluten-free rolled oats

1 cup unsweetened almond milk or any milk of choice

½ cup canned pumpkin purée

1 tablespoon chia seeds

1 tablespoon maple syrup or honey, optional

½ teaspoon ground cinnamon

¼ teaspoon ground nutmeg

¼ teaspoon ground ginger

Pinch of salt

SERVING OPTIONS

Chopped pecans

Toasted pumpkin seeds

Sliced banana

Dried cranberries or cherries

Toasted coconut flakes

1 In a small saucepan over medium heat, add the rolled oats and almond milk.

2 Stirring occasionally, bring the mixture to a gentle boil.

3 Once it starts boiling, reduce the heat to low, and add in the pumpkin purée, chia seeds, maple syrup (if using), cinnamon, nutmeg, ginger, and a pinch of salt. Stir to combine.

4 Simmer the oatmeal for about 5 minutes or until it has reached your desired consistency.

5 Remove the saucepan from the heat and let the oatmeal cool slightly.

6 Serve the pumpkin oatmeal in bowls and serve as desired with your favorite toppings, such as chopped nuts, seeds, sliced banana, dried fruits, or coconut flakes.

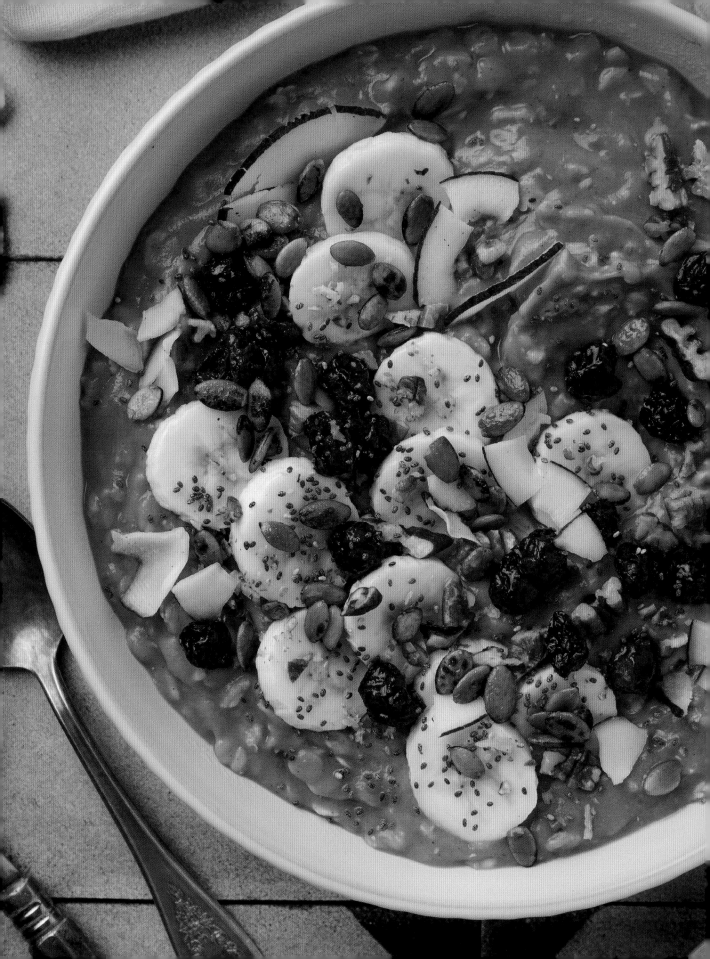

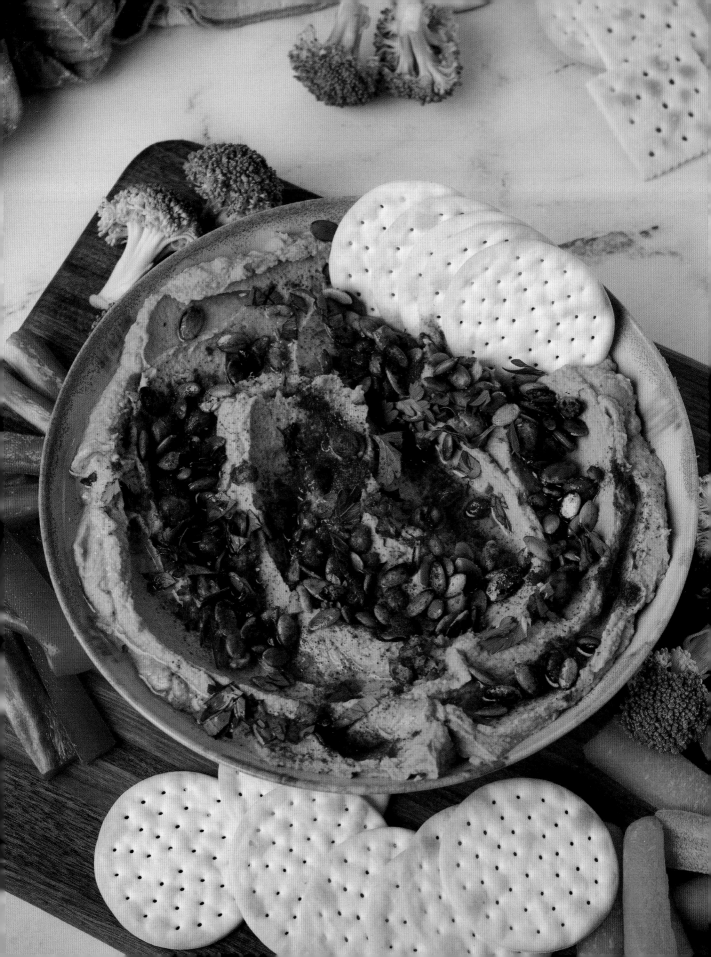

PUMPKIN HUMMUS

Rachael: This week we are going to incorporate some recipes that might add a little pep to your step and some much-needed energy to carry you to the finish line. This pumpkin hummus will do just that! Because hummus is made from chickpeas that are high in protein and have a low glycemic index, this snack will digest more slowly than other foods, giving you the midday power boost that we all know you need.

SERVINGS: 4–6	PREP TIME: 15 MINUTES	TOTAL TIME: 15 MINUTES

1 cup canned pumpkin purée
2 garlic cloves, minced
3 tablespoons tahini
Juice of 1 lemon
2 tablespoons extra-virgin olive oil
2 teaspoons ground cumin
1 teaspoon ground cinnamon
½ teaspoon ground ginger
Pinch salt
1 (15-ounce/425g) can chickpeas
  (garbanzo beans), drained and rinsed

SERVING OPTIONS
Extra-virgin olive oil
Toasted pumpkin seeds
Chopped fresh parsley
Gluten-free crackers
Sliced vegetables

1 In a food processor, combine the pumpkin purée, garlic, tahini, lemon juice, olive oil, cumin, cinnamon, ginger, and salt. Whip ingredients until well blended.

2 Add the drained chickpeas to the mixture in batches, allowing them to blend fully before adding more, until all have been incorporated. Scrape down the sides of the food processor as needed to ensure everything is well blended and smooth. If the hummus seems too thick, you can add a little water, one tablespoon at a time, until you reach your desired consistency.

3 Taste the hummus and adjust the seasoning to your taste, adding more salt or lemon juice if needed. Once the hummus is smooth and seasoned to your liking, transfer it to a serving bowl.

4 Drizzle a little extra-virgin olive oil over the top of the hummus and sprinkle with toasted pumpkin seeds and chopped fresh parsley for garnish, if desired.

5 Serve the pumpkin hummus with your favorite gluten-free crackers or sliced vegetables, or use it as a spread on sandwiches or wraps.

Notes *Ensure pumpkin purée, not pumpkin-pie filling, is used for this recipe. Removing the skins from the chickpeas makes for a creamier hummus. To do this, soak the drained chickpeas in water and rub them vigorously until the skins come off and float, then drain again.*

WATERMELON POUTINE
WITH DATE SYRUP & STRAWBERRY DIP

Rachael: Is this not the cutest way to prepare watermelon? If you don't have a crinkle cutter, I think it's an unnecessary but also very necessary purchase. Yes, you can cut the watermelon into fries without it, and it will taste the same, but do it for the aesthetic! And because it's week 40 and dates are suggested to help ease labor pains, we added a date syrup to help slide that baby out.

SERVINGS: 4	PREP TIME: 15 MINUTES	TOTAL TIME: 35 MINUTES

1 small seedless watermelon, rind removed
¼ cup feta cheese
¼ cup chopped fresh mint leaves

FOR THE DATE SYRUP
1 cup pitted dates
¾ cup of reserved date water
1 teaspoon lemon juice
Pinch of salt

FOR THE STRAWBERRY DIP
4 fresh strawberries, rinsed and hulled
½ cup plain yogurt (we prefer cashew yogurt)
1 tablespoon honey

1 **Prepare the strawberry dip** by combining all the ingredients in a blender and blending on high until smooth. Pour the dip into a small bowl or ramekin, cover, and refrigerate for at least 30 minutes.

2 Use a sharp knife to slice the watermelon into ¼- to ½-inch-thick (6mm-1.25cm) sticks, resembling traditional fries. You can also use a crinkle cutter tool to add some texture. Set aside on a paper towel to drain.

3 **Make the date syrup.** Soak the dates in 1 cup of hot water for 30 minutes. Drain the dates, reserving the soaking water. In a blender or food processor, combine the dates and ¾ cup of the reserved date water. Blend until smooth and creamy, adding more water, a tablespoon at a time, if needed to reach your desired consistency. The syrup should be thick but still pourable.

4 **Assemble the watermelon poutine.** Arrange the watermelon fries on a serving platter. Drizzle the date syrup generously over the watermelon. Sprinkle crumbled feta cheese and chopped mint over the watermelon fries. Serve with the chilled strawberry dip on the side.

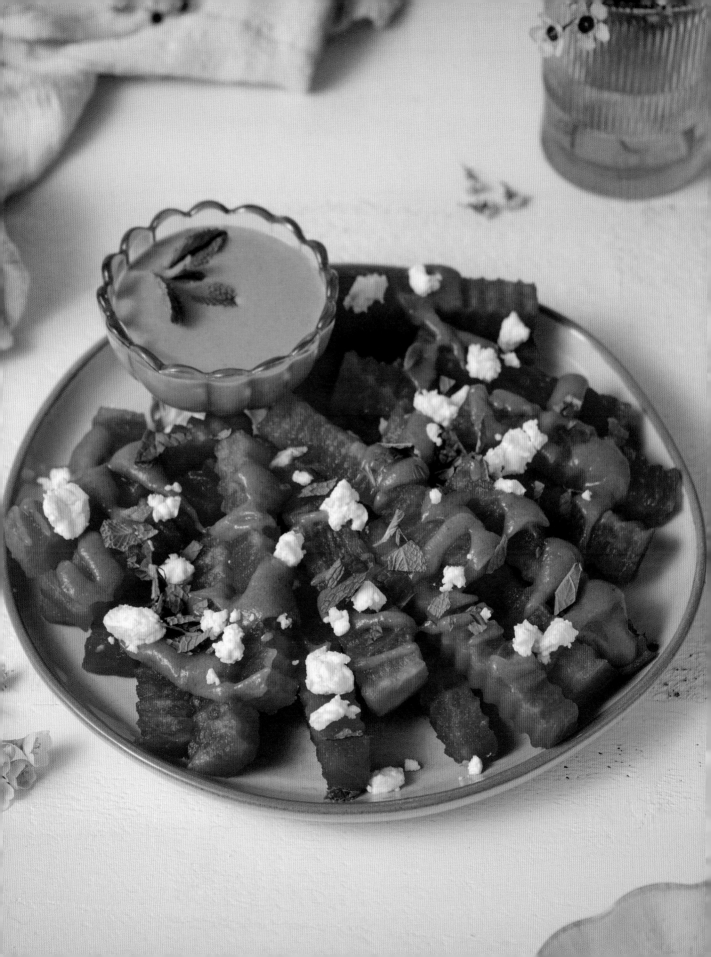

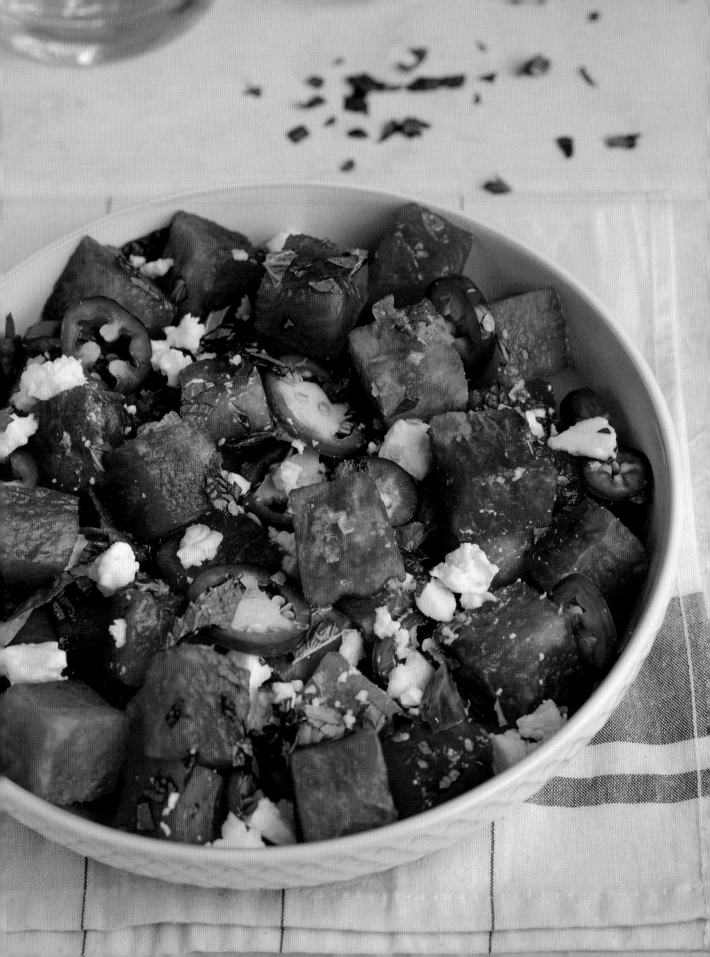

WATERMELON SALAD
WITH JALAPEÑO & LIME

Rachael: Welcome, friend! You have arrived at your destination! A few weeks ago, you may have been anxious as the due date was approaching. I sure was, but I hope at this point you feel a sense of peace within you. At any moment, you will get to have your first "meet and greet" with this little angel of yours, and it's one of the greatest feelings you will ever experience. Let's keep this week simple with a watermelon salad that includes mint, basil, and lime, and only takes a few minutes to prepare. You have a whole lot of other things that need your preparation at this point, but we just want to thank you for letting us be a part of the journey.

SERVINGS: 2–4	PREP TIME: 10 MINUTES	TOTAL TIME: 40 MINUTES

4 cups cubed seedless watermelon, rind removed

1 jalapeño, thinly sliced, seeds removed if less heat desired

¼ cup chopped fresh mint leaves

¼ cup chopped fresh basil leaves

Juice of 1 lime

1 tablespoon honey

Crumbled feta cheese or goat cheese, optional

1 teaspoon flaky sea salt

1　Place the watermelon cubes in a large mixing bowl.

2　Add the jalapeño slices, mint, and basil.

3　Squeeze the lime juice over the watermelon and herbs.

4　Drizzle honey over the salad for a touch of sweetness.

5　Gently toss all the ingredients together until the watermelon cubes are evenly coated.

6　If using feta cheese, sprinkle it over the top of the salad for added creaminess and flavor.

7　Cover the bowl and refrigerate the watermelon salad for at least 30 minutes to allow the flavors to meld and the salad to chill.

8　Right before serving, sprinkle flaky sea salt over the top.

— week 40 —

WATERMELON "CAKE"
WITH WHIPPED COCONUT TOPPING

Rachael: We have a very special birthday to celebrate this week, and you can't celebrate a birthday without some cake! These last few weeks will live vividly in your memory. You have faced a lot of challenges to get to this point, but there has also been a lot of love and happiness. Our hope is that you take this last recipe, a watermelon "cake," and truly relish in the joys and sweetness of life.

SERVINGS: 2–4	PREP TIME: 15 MINUTES	TOTAL TIME: 45 MINUTES

1 large seedless watermelon, washed and dried
Fresh berries, such as strawberries, blueberries, raspberries
Fresh mint leaves
Edible flowers

FOR THE WHIPPED TOPPING
1 (14-ounce/397g) can full-fat coconut milk, chilled in the fridge overnight
1 tablespoon honey or maple syrup, optional
1 teaspoon vanilla extract

1 Place a large metal mixing bowl and beaters in the freezer for about 10 minutes to chill.

2 Using a sharp knife, slice off the top and bottom ends of the watermelon to create a stable base. Stand the watermelon upright on one of the cut ends. Carefully slice away the rind, following the natural curve of the watermelon, and then cut it lengthwise into 3 to 4 even slices of watermelon to make the "cake" layers.

3 **Prepare the whipped topping.** Open the chilled can of coconut milk and scoop out the thick coconut cream that has risen to the top, leaving the watery liquid behind. (Reserve it for another use.)

4 Place the coconut cream in the chilled bowl. Add the honey, if using, and vanilla extract.

5 Using a hand mixer or stand mixer, beat the coconut cream on high speed until it becomes thick and fluffy, resembling whipped cream. This may take 2 to 3 minutes.

6 Place one layer of the watermelon on a serving platter or cake stand.

7 Spread a layer of the whipped coconut cream evenly over the top of the watermelon layer, then place the next watermelon layer on top of the cream.

8 Repeat this process with the remaining layers of watermelon and whipped coconut cream, stacking them on top of each other ending with a layer of whipped cream on top.

9 Garnish the top of the cake with fresh berries, mint, or edible flowers.

10 Place the assembled watermelon cake in the fridge for at least 30 minutes to chill before cutting and serving.

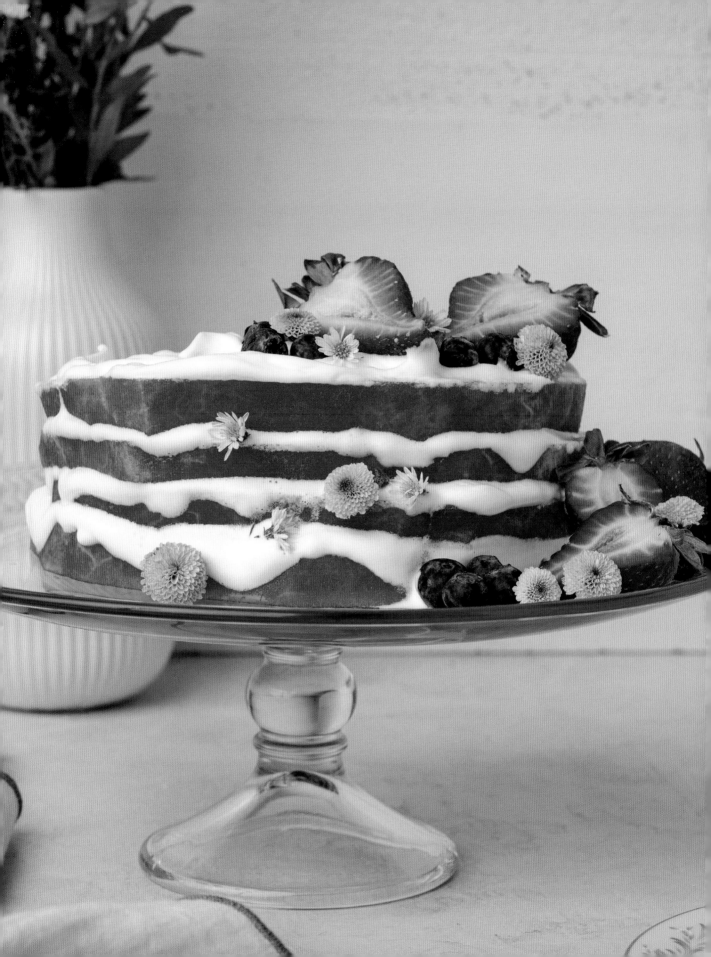

FOURTH TRIMESTER

As I write this, I am currently four weeks into my own fourth trimester. Yes, you read that correct—the fourth trimester. It's 6:49 a.m., and I just finished our first feed of the day. Now, I normally spend the next hour cuddling my baby while she sleeps because these moments are so fleeting. But today, instead of cuddles, I'm in our living room writing this letter to you as encouragement and support for the next twelve weeks, as I too am in the thick of it.

The moment your baby enters this world, you enter the fourth trimester. While most people focus on the baby during this time, I want to focus on you and what you just accomplished. Your birth story will be one of the most empowering tales you ever get to tell: one that involves blood, sweat, and tears and ends with meeting the love of your life. Birth is no small feat, and neither is the recovery process. Give yourself grace and be okay with slowing down. Your days will now be dictated by naps, diapers, and feedings, but gratitude will occupy more space than exhaustion. Whether this is your first rodeo or not, there is a learning curve for us all. Each birth brings its own set of beautiful challenges and a new chapter in your family's life.

 Give yourself compassion during this time. There is so much healing to be done—not only physically, but mentally too. I feel extra compelled to reiterate this statement because I too am four weeks into the mom guilt, struggling to balance work life, family life, and the mental exhaustion of it all. Even though I feel I am falling short in so many facets of my life right now, I have to constantly remind myself that I am not meant to function at 100 percent. I have this beautiful life right now. I am someone's entire world. The rest of my world will have to wait.

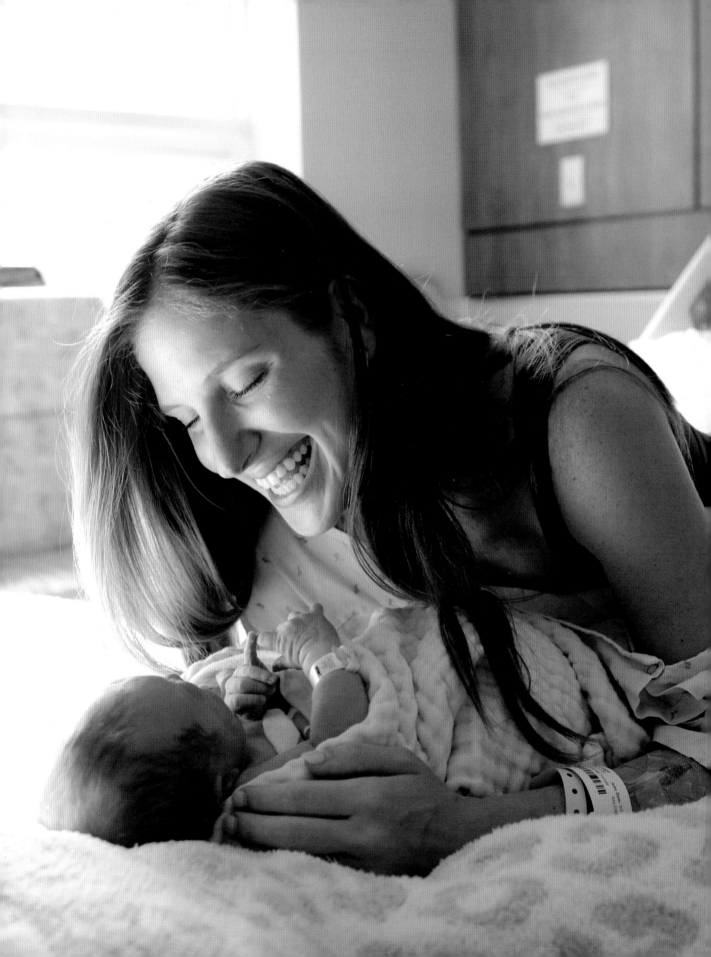

INDEX

A

apple (week 15)
Apple Nachos, 78
Apple, Sweet Potato & Sausage Breakfast Skillet, 81
Green Apple BLT, 82
Grilled Endive with Fig, Apple & Walnut Salad, 94
Rhubarb, Apple & Almond Cobbler, 226
Arugula & Fig Pizza, 49
avocado (week 16)
Avocado Huevos Rancheros Toast, 85
Fish Tacos with Grapefruit Avocado Salsa, 125
Jicama Fries with Creamy Avocado Dipping Sauce, 150
Mediterranean Chickpea Avocado Boats, Three Ways, 89
Mint Chocolate Chip Avocado Ice Cream, 86

B

baby size chart, 22–23
Baked Kale Frittata, 230
banana (week 23)
Banana French Toast, 130
Banana Recovery Smoothie, 133
Banana Sushi, Three Ways, 129
Fig & Banana Smoothie, 53
Mint Chocolate Chip Avocado Ice Cream, 86
beef
Mango & Beef Skewers, 105
Sweet Potato Shepherd's Pie, 117
beverages
Banana Recovery Smoothie, 133
Cucumber Margarita Mocktail, 170
Fig & Banana Smoothie, 53
Piña Colada, 182
Pink Drink, 113
Raspberry Ginger Tea, 37
Spicy Margarita Mocktail, 57
Blackened Cauliflower with Citrus Herb Salad, 201
blueberry (week 8)
Blueberry & Chipotle Chicken, 34
Blueberry Skillet Pancake, 30
bowls
Chipotle Butternut Squash & Plantain Bowl with Spicy Cranberry Sauce, 210–211

Dragon Fruit & Shrimp Poke Bowl with Forbidden Black Rice, 110
Mango Smoothie Bowl, 106
breads
Avocado Huevos Rancheros Toast, 85
Fig & Walnut Cornbread, 50
Yogurt Toast with Cantaloupe Ribbons, 218
breakfast
Apple, Sweet Potato & Sausage Breakfast Skillet, 81
Banana French Toast, 130
Blueberry Skillet Pancake, 30
Key Lime Pie Overnight Oats, 54
Lemon, Blueberry & Lavender Overnight Oats, 33
Pumpkin French Toast Casserole, 237
Raspberry Marmalade Breakfast Sliders, 41
Broiled Plantain Ice Cream Split, 186
Brussels sprouts, Cherry-Balsamic Brussels Sprouts, 45
butternut squash (week 35)
Butternut Squash Risotto, 214
Chipotle Butternut Squash & Plantain Bowl with Spicy Cranberry Sauce, 210–211
Roasted Butternut Squash Soup, 209
Sheet Pan Butternut Squash & Lemon Cashew Yogurt, 213

C

cabbage (week 32)
Cabbage Stir-Fry, 193
Stuffed Cabbage Rolls with Tomato Sauce, 194
Candied Grapefruit Parfait, 122
cantaloupe (week 36)
Cantaloupe & Herb Salad with Chili-Lime Vinaigrette, 221
Grilled Prosciutto-Wrapped Cantaloupe with Honey, 217
Yogurt Toast with Cantaloupe Ribbons, 218
carrot (week 24)
Carrot Fries with Dipping Sauce, 138
Carrot Ribbon Salad, 134
Ginger Carrot Soup, 137
cauliflower (week 33)
Blackened Cauliflower with Citrus Herb Salad, 201
Cauliflower Curry, 198
Cauliflower Steak with Chimichurri, 197

Charred-Corn Maque Choux, 141
Charred Corn & Onion Chowder, 142
cheese, Grilled Peach-Basil Goat Cheese Sandwiches, 66
cherry (week 10)
Cherry-Balsamic Brussels Sprouts, 45
Cherry & Rosemary Chicken, 46
Cherry Vinaigrette Wedge Salad, 42
chicken
Blueberry & Chipotle Chicken, 34
Cherry & Rosemary Chicken, 46
Cilantro-Lime Coconut Chicken, 58
Coconut Curry Chicken & Vegetables, 178
Jibarito Chicken Sandwich with Garlic Sauce, 185
Raspberry Dijon Chicken, 38
Rhubarb-Glazed Chicken Wings, 222
Sonoma Chicken Salad, 161
chickpeas, Mediterranean Chickpea Avocado Boats, Three Ways, 89
Chipotle Butternut Squash & Plantain Bowl with Spicy Cranberry Sauce, 210–211
chocolate
Banana Sushi, Three Ways, 129
Chocolate-Covered Dried Mangos, 109
Mint Chocolate Chip Avocado Ice Cream, 86
Pomegranate & Dark Chocolate Bites, 101
Cilantro-Lime Coconut Chicken, 58
coconut (week 30)
Coconut-Crusted Seafood with Mango Salsa, 181
Coconut Curry Chicken & Vegetables, 178
Piña Colada, 182
cookies, Peach-Cobbler Cookies, 70
corn (week 25)
Charred-Corn Maque Choux, 141
Charred Corn & Onion Chowder, 142
Thai Street-Corn Salad, 145
cranberry, Chipotle Butternut Squash & Plantain Bowl with Spicy Cranberry Sauce, 210–211
Crispy Eggplant Tacos, 173
Cuban Slaw, 190
cucumber (week 28)
Cucumber Margarita Mocktail, 170
Cucumber Salsa Verde with Shrimp, 166
Cucumber Tahini Salad, 165
Mediterranean Cucumber Wrap, 169

D

dragon fruit (week 20)
    Dragon Fruit Kabobs, 114
    Dragon Fruit & Shrimp Poke Bowl
        with Forbidden Black Rice, 110
duck, Crispy Duck Breast with Rhubarb
    Chutney, 225

E

eggplant (week 29)
    Crispy Eggplant Tacos, 173
    Eggplant Dip, 174
    Eggplant Lasagna Stack, 177
eggs
    Apple, Sweet Potato & Sausage
        Breakfast Skillet, 81
    Avocado Huevos Rancheros Toast,
        85
    Raspberry Marmalade Breakfast
        Sliders, 41
endive (week 17)
    Endive Cups, Three Ways, 90
    Endive Stir-Fry with Vegetables &
        Ground Turkey, 93
    Grilled Endive with Fig, Apple &
        Walnut Salad, 94

F

Fall-Winter Pear Salad, 77
fertility journey, 14–19
fig (week 11)
    Arugula & Fig Pizza, 49
    Fig & Banana Smoothie, 53
    Fig & Walnut Cornbread, 50
    Grilled Endive with Fig, Apple &
        Walnut Salad, 94
first trimester, 25–29
    milestones, 26
    preparation, 29
    symptoms, 26
    weeks 8 through 12, 30–58
        week 8 (blueberry), 30–35
        week 9 (raspberry), 37–41
        week 10 (cherry), 42–46
        week 11 (fig), 49–53
        week 12 (lime), 54–58
Fish Tacos with Grapefruit Avocado
    Salsa, 125
fourth trimester, 248
fruit. See specific fruit

G

Ginger Carrot Soup, 137
grains, Pomegranate Quinoa Salad, 97
grapefruit (week 22)
    Candied Grapefruit Parfait, 122
    Fish Tacos with Grapefruit Avocado
        Salsa, 125
    Rosemary Grapefruit Granita, 126
grapes (week 27)
    Grape Harvest Crisp, 162
    Roasted Grape & Red Onion Pork,
        158
Green Apple BLT, 82
Grilled Endive with Fig, Apple &
    Walnut Salad, 94
Grilled Peach-Basil Goat Cheese
    Sandwiches, 66
Grilled Prosciutto-Wrapped
    Cantaloupe with Honey, 217

H–I

ham
    Grilled Prosciutto-Wrapped
        Cantaloupe with Honey, 217
    Pear & Prosciutto Poppers, 74
hummus, Pumpkin Hummus, 241

ice cream
    Broiled Plantain Ice Cream Split, 186
    Mint Chocolate Chip Avocado Ice
        Cream, 86

J

jicama (week 26)
    Jicama Ceviche with Jicama Chips,
        146
    Jicama Fries with Creamy Avocado
        Dipping Sauce, 150
    Sautéed Shrimp with Jicama &
        Cilantro Slaw, 149

K

kale (week 38)
    Baked Kale Frittata, 230
    Kale Caesar Salad, 229
    Kale Chips, Four Ways, 233
Key Lime Pie Overnight Oats, 54

L

lamb
    Lamb with Peach & Mint Pesto, 69
    Sweet Potato Shepherd's Pie, 117
lemon
    Lemonade with Pomegranate &
        Rosemary Ice Cubes, 98
    Lemon, Blueberry & Lavender
        Overnight Oats, 33
lime (week 12)
    Cilantro-Lime Coconut Chicken, 58
    Key Lime Pie Overnight Oats, 54

M

mango (week 19)
    Chocolate-Covered Dried Mangos,
        109
    Coconut-Crusted Seafood with
        Mango Salsa, 181
    Mango & Beef Skewers, 105
    Mango Smoothie Bowl, 106
Meals She Eats, 14, 21, 81
Mediterranean Chickpea Avocado
    Boats, Three Ways, 89
Mediterranean Cucumber Wrap, 169
Mint Chocolate Chip Avocado Ice
    Cream, 86

N

nachos, Apple Nachos, 78
nuts
    Fig & Walnut Cornbread, 50
    Grilled Endive with Fig, Apple &
        Walnut Salad, 94
    Rhubarb, Apple & Almond Cobbler,
        226
    Sheet Pan Butternut Squash &
        Lemon Cashew Yogurt, 213

O

oats
    Grape Harvest Crisp, 162
    Key Lime Pie Overnight Oats, 54
    Pumpkin Oatmeal, 238
onion
    Charred Corn & Onion Chowder,
        142
    Roasted Grape & Red Onion Pork,
        158

P–Q

PCOS, 14

peach (week 13)
    Grilled Peach-Basil Goat Cheese Sandwiches, 66
    Peach-Cobbler Cookies, 70

pear (week 14)
    Fall-Winter Pear Salad, 77
    Pear-Mostarda Pork Chops, 73
    Pear & Prosciutto Poppers, 74

Piña Colada, 182

pineapple (week 34)
    Pineapple Whip, 202
    Shrimp Fried Rice in a Pineapple Boat, 205
    Slow-Cooker Pineapple Pulled Pork, Three Ways, 206–207

Pink Drink, 113

pizza, Arugula & Fig Pizza, 49

plantain (week 31)
    Broiled Plantain Ice Cream Split, 186
    Tostones with Herb Dipping Sauce, 189

pomegranate (week 18)
    Lemonade with Pomegranate & Rosemary Ice Cubes, 98
    Pomegranate & Dark Chocolate Bites, 101
    Pomegranate Quinoa Salad, 97
    Pomegranate-Stuffed Sweet Potatoes, 102

pork
    Pear-Mostarda Pork Chops, 73
    Roasted Grape & Red Onion Pork, 158
    Slow-Cooker Pineapple Pulled Pork, Three Ways, 206–207

poultry
    Blueberry & Chipotle Chicken, 34
    Cherry & Rosemary Chicken, 46
    Cilantro-Lime Coconut Chicken, 58
    Coconut Curry Chicken & Vegetables, 178
    Crispy Duck Breast with Rhubarb Chutney, 225
    Jibarito Chicken Sandwich with Garlic Sauce, 185
    Raspberry Dijon Chicken, 38
    Rhubarb-Glazed Chicken Wings, 222
    Sonoma Chicken Salad, 161

pumpkin (week 39)
    Pumpkin French Toast Casserole, 237
    Pumpkin Hummus, 241
    Pumpkin Oatmeal, 238
    Savory Pumpkin Pasta Sauce, 234

quinoa, Pomegranate Quinoa Salad, 97

R

raspberry (week 9)
    Raspberry Dijon Chicken, 38
    Raspberry Ginger Tea, 37
    Raspberry Marmalade Breakfast Sliders, 41

rhubarb (week 37)
    Crispy Duck Breast with Rhubarb Chutney, 225
    Rhubarb, Apple & Almond Cobbler, 226
    Rhubarb-Glazed Chicken Wings, 222

rice
    Dragon Fruit & Shrimp Poke Bowl with Forbidden Black Rice, 110
    Shrimp Fried Rice in a Pineapple Boat, 205

Roasted Butternut Squash Soup, 209

Roasted Grape & Red Onion Pork, 158

Rosemary Grapefruit Granita, 126

Rosie, 18–19

S

salads
    Blackened Cauliflower with Citrus Herb Salad, 201
    Cantaloupe & Herb Salad with Chili-Lime Vinaigrette, 221
    Carrot Ribbon Salad, 134
    Cherry Vinaigrette Wedge Salad, 42
    Fall-Winter Pear Salad, 77
    Grilled Endive with Fig, Apple & Walnut Salad, 94
    Kale Caesar Salad, 229
    Pomegranate Quinoa Salad, 97
    Sonoma Chicken Salad, 161
    Thai Street-Corn Salad, 145
    Watermelon Salad with Jalapeño & Lime, 245

salsa
    Coconut-Crusted Seafood with Mango Salsa, 181
    Cucumber Salsa Verde with Shrimp, 166
    Fish Tacos with Grapefruit Avocado Salsa, 125

sandwiches
    Green Apple BLT, 82
    Grilled Peach-Basil Goat Cheese Sandwiches, 66
    Jibarito Chicken Sandwich with Garlic Sauce, 185
    Raspberry Marmalade Breakfast Sliders, 41

sausage, Apple, Sweet Potato & Sausage Breakfast Skillet, 81

Sautéed Shrimp with Jicama & Cilantro Slaw, 149

Savory Pumpkin Pasta Sauce, 234

seafood
    Coconut-Crusted Seafood with Mango Salsa, 181
    Cucumber Salsa Verde with Shrimp, 166
    Dragon Fruit & Shrimp Poke Bowl with Forbidden Black Rice, 110
    Fish Tacos with Grapefruit Avocado Salsa, 125
    Sautéed Shrimp with Jicama & Cilantro Slaw, 149
    Shrimp Fried Rice in a Pineapple Boat, 205

second trimester, 61–150
    milestones, 62
    preparation, 65
    symptoms, 62
    weeks 13 through 26, 66–150
        week 13 (peach), 66–70
        week 14 (pear), 73–77
        week 15 (apple), 78–82
        week 16 (avocado), 85–89
        week 17 (endive), 90–94
        week 18 (pomegranate), 97–102
        week 19 (mango), 105–109
        week 20 (dragon fruit), 110–114
        week 21 (sweet potato), 117–121
        week 22 (grapefruit), 122–126
        week 23 (banana), 129–133
        week 24 (carrot), 134–138
        week 25 (corn), 141–145
        week 26 (jicama), 146–150

Sheet Pan Butternut Squash & Lemon Cashew Yogurt, 213

shrimp
    Cucumber Salsa Verde with Shrimp, 166
    Dragon Fruit & Shrimp Poke Bowl with Forbidden Black Rice, 110
    Sautéed Shrimp with Jicama & Cilantro Slaw, 149
    Shrimp Fried Rice in a Pineapple Boat, 205

slaw
    Cuban Slaw, 190
    Sautéed Shrimp with Jicama & Cilantro Slaw, 149

Slow-Cooker Pineapple Pulled Pork, Three Ways, 206–207

smoothies
    Banana Recovery Smoothie, 133
    Fig & Banana Smoothie, 53

Sonoma Chicken Salad, 161

soups
    Charred Corn & Onion Chowder, 142
    Ginger Carrot Soup, 137
    Roasted Butternut Squash Soup, 209

Spicy Margarita Mocktail, 57
squash, butternut (week 35)
    Butternut Squash Risotto, 214
    Chipotle Butternut Squash &
        Plantain Bowl with Spicy
        Cranberry Sauce, 210–211
    Roasted Butternut Squash Soup,
        209
    Sheet Pan Butternut Squash &
        Lemon Cashew Yogurt, 213
stir-fry
    Cabbage Stir-Fry, 193
    Endive Stir-Fry with Vegetables &
        Ground Turkey, 93
Stuffed Cabbage Rolls with Tomato
    Sauce, 194
Sullivan, Lenore, 19
sweet potato (week 21)
    Apple, Sweet Potato & Sausage
        Breakfast Skillet, 81
    Pomegranate-Stuffed Sweet
        Potatoes, 102
    Sweet Potato Gnocchi with
        Roasted Onion & Coconut Sauce,
        118–119
    Sweet Potato Shepherd's Pie, 117
    Sweet Potato Toast, Three Ways, 121

T–U–V

tacos
    Crispy Eggplant Tacos, 173
    Fish Tacos with Grapefruit Avocado
        Salsa, 125
tahini, Cucumber Tahini Salad, 165
Thai Street-Corn Salad, 145
third trimester, 153–246
    milestones, 154
    preparation, 157
    symptoms, 154
    weeks 27 through 40, 158–246
        week 27 (grapes), 158–162
        week 28 (cucumber), 165–170
        week 29 (eggplant), 173–177
        week 30 (coconut), 178–182
        week 31 (plantain), 185–189
        week 32 (cabbage), 190–194
        week 33 (cauliflower), 197–201
        week 34 (pineapple), 202–207
        week 35 (butternut squash),
            209–214
        week 36 (cantaloupe), 217–221
        week 37 (rhubarb), 222–226
        week 38 (kale), 229–233
        week 39 (pumpkin), 234–241
        week 40 (watermelon), 242–246
Tostones with Herb Dipping Sauce,
    189
turkey, Endive Stir-Fry with Vegetables
    & Ground Turkey, 93

vegetables. See specific vegetable

W–X–Y–Z

watermelon (week 40)
    Watermelon "Cake" with Whipped
        Coconut Frosting, 246
    Watermelon Poutine with Date
        Syrup & Strawberry Dip, 242
    Watermelon Salad with Jalapeño &
        Lime, 245
week 8 (blueberry), 30–35
    Blueberry & Chipotle Chicken, 34
    Blueberry Skillet Pancake, 30
    Lemon, Blueberry & Lavender
        Overnight Oats, 33
week 9 (raspberry), 37–41
    Raspberry Dijon Chicken, 38
    Raspberry Ginger Tea, 37
    Raspberry Marmalade Breakfast
        Sliders, 41
week 10 (cherry), 42–46
    Cherry-Balsamic Brussels Sprouts,
        45
    Cherry & Rosemary Chicken, 46
    Cherry Vinaigrette Wedge Salad, 42
week 11 (fig), 49–53
    Arugula & Fig Pizza, 49
    Fig & Banana Smoothie, 53
    Fig & Walnut Cornbread, 50
week 12 (lime), 54–58
    Cilantro-Lime Coconut Chicken, 58
    Key Lime Pie Overnight Oats, 54
    Spicy Margarita Mocktail, 57
week 13 (peach), 66–70
    Grilled Peach-Basil Goat Cheese
        Sandwiches, 66
    Lamb with Peach & Mint Pesto, 69
    Peach-Cobbler Cookies, 70
week 14 (pear), 73–77
    Fall-Winter Pear Salad, 77
    Pear-Mostarda Pork Chops, 73
    Pear & Prosciutto Poppers, 74
week 15 (apple), 78–82
    Apple Nachos, 78
    Apple, Sweet Potato & Sausage
        Breakfast Skillet, 81
    Green Apple BLT, 82
week 16 (avocado), 85–89
    Avocado Huevos Rancheros Toast,
        85
    Mediterranean Chickpea Avocado
        Boats, Three Ways, 89
    Mint Chocolate Chip Avocado Ice
        Cream, 86
week 17 (endive), 90–94
    Endive Cups, Three Ways, 90
    Endive Stir-Fry with Vegetables &
        Ground Turkey, 93
    Grilled Endive with Fig, Apple &
        Walnut Salad, 94
week 18 (pomegranate), 97–102
    Lemonade with Pomegranate &
        Rosemary Ice Cubes, 98
    Pomegranate & Dark Chocolate
        Bites, 101
    Pomegranate Quinoa Salad, 97
    Pomegranate-Stuffed Sweet
        Potatoes, 102
week 19 (mango), 105–109
    Chocolate-Covered Dried Mangos,
        109
    Mango & Beef Skewers, 105
    Mango Smoothie Bowl, 106
week 20 (dragon fruit), 110–114
    Dragon Fruit Kabobs, 114
    Dragon Fruit & Shrimp Poke Bowl
        with Forbidden Black Rice, 110
    Pink Drink, 113
week 21 (sweet potato), 117–121
    Sweet Potato Gnocchi with
        Roasted Onion & Coconut Sauce,
        118–119
    Sweet Potato Shepherd's Pie, 117
    Sweet Potato Toast, Three Ways, 121
week 22 (grapefruit), 122–126
    Candied Grapefruit Parfait, 122
    Fish Tacos with Grapefruit Avocado
        Salsa, 125
    Rosemary Grapefruit Granita, 126
week 23 (banana), 129–133
    Banana French Toast, 130
    Banana Recovery Smoothie, 133
    Banana Sushi, Three Ways, 129
week 24 (carrot), 134–138
    Carrot Fries with Dipping Sauce, 138
    Carrot Ribbon Salad, 134
    Ginger Carrot Soup, 137
week 25 (corn), 141–145
    Charred-Corn Maque Choux, 141
    Charred Corn & Onion Chowder,
        142
    Thai Street-Corn Salad, 145
week 26 (jicama), 146–150
    Jicama Ceviche with Jicama Chips,
        146
    Jicama Fries with Creamy Avocado
        Dipping Sauce, 150
    Sautéed Shrimp with Jicama &
        Cilantro Slaw, 149
week 27 (grapes), 158–162
    Grape Harvest Crisp, 162
    Roasted Grape & Red Onion Pork,
        158
    Sonoma Chicken Salad, 161
week 28 (cucumber), 165–170
    Cucumber Margarita Mocktail, 170
    Cucumber Salsa Verde with Shrimp,
        166
    Cucumber Tahini Salad, 165
    Mediterranean Cucumber Wrap, 169
week 29 (eggplant), 173–177
    Crispy Eggplant Tacos, 173
    Eggplant Dip, 174
    Eggplant Lasagna Stack, 177

week 30 (coconut), 178–182
  Coconut-Crusted Seafood with
    Mango Salsa, 181
  Coconut Curry Chicken &
    Vegetables, 178
  Piña Colada, 182
week 31 (plantain), 185–189
  Broiled Plantain Ice Cream Split, 186
  Jibarito Chicken Sandwich with
    Garlic Sauce, 185
  Tostones with Herb Dipping Sauce,
    189
week 32 (cabbage), 190–194
  Cabbage Stir-Fry, 193
  Cuban Slaw, 190
  Stuffed Cabbage Rolls with Tomato
    Sauce, 194
week 33 (cauliflower), 197–201
  Blackened Cauliflower with Citrus
    Herb Salad, 201
  Cauliflower Curry, 198
  Cauliflower Steak with Chimichurri,
    197
week 34 (pineapple), 202–207
  Pineapple Whip, 202
  Shrimp Fried Rice in a Pineapple
    Boat, 205
  Slow-Cooker Pineapple Pulled Pork,
    Three Ways, 206–207
week 35 (butternut squash), 209–214
  Butternut Squash Risotto, 214
  Chipotle Butternut Squash &
    Plantain Bowl with Spicy
    Cranberry Sauce, 210–211
  Roasted Butternut Squash Soup,
    209
  Sheet Pan Butternut Squash &
    Lemon Cashew Yogurt, 213
week 36 (cantaloupe), 217–221
  Cantaloupe & Herb Salad with
    Chili-Lime Vinaigrette, 221
  Grilled Prosciutto-Wrapped
    Cantaloupe with Honey, 217
  Yogurt Toast with Cantaloupe
    Ribbons, 218
week 37 (rhubarb), 222–226
  Crispy Duck Breast with Rhubarb
    Chutney, 225
  Rhubarb, Apple & Almond Cobbler,
    226
  Rhubarb-Glazed Chicken Wings,
    222
week 38 (kale), 229–233
  Baked Kale Frittata, 230
  Kale Caesar Salad, 229
  Kale Chips, Four Ways, 233

week 39 (pumpkin), 234–241
  Pumpkin French Toast
    Casserole, 237
  Pumpkin Hummus, 241
  Pumpkin Oatmeal, 238
  Savory Pumpkin Pasta Sauce,
    234
week 40 (watermelon), 242–246
  Watermelon "Cake" with
    Whipped Coconut Frosting,
    246
  Watermelon Poutine with Date
    Syrup & Strawberry Dip, 242
  Watermelon Salad with
    Jalapeño & Lime, 245
wraps, Mediterranean Cucumber
  Wrap, 169

yogurt
  Sheet Pan Butternut Squash &
    Lemon Cashew Yogurt, 213
  Yogurt Toast with Cantaloupe
    Ribbons, 218

ACKNOWLEDGMENTS

Sutton: You don't even know it, but your pure love and natural optimism in life really helped us get this book over the finish line. Writing this book while grieving, raising a toddler, and in the middle of a pregnancy was no small task. You are an inspiration to us, Mom and Dad, that we will truly never be able to put into words. Thank you for being the amazing person you are. We love you so much, Sutton.

Jason "Boss Man" Allen: Thank you for being an amazing friend and an incredible chef. It's not easy finding someone who can cook gluten- and dairy-free with ease like yourself. These recipes would not have been able to be pulled together without your help.

Santino: The quarterback of the team! You work ethic, creativity, and being able to wear 10 hats a day is a THE reason why we are so proud of this book and our vision was able to come to life. Special shoutout to Jen for being the rock you are, keeping Santino in line, and not murdering him for the crazy amount of time and travel he put into bringing this to life.

Michael and Hannah Jones: Legends! From your pep talks to your unwavering belief in us, you are the best people we could ever ask to have in our corner. The list of ways you support us and make dreams become reality could be an entire book of its own. When your management team becomes family, you know you have something special.

The Duo of Bailey and Sierra: Thank you putting out our fires, keeping us on task, adjusting our schedules, and overall being ROCK STARS. You take our chaos and give it harmony. We are lucky and grateful to have you on our team.

Glam Squad Denise Ferguson & Shannon Schickel: If there is one thing we can bet the house on, it is hair and make-up will be flawless. Not only are you both extremely skilled in your profession, you also have amazing personalities that are contagious. You have the gift of making people feel beautiful, and it has nothing to do with the makeup or hairspray—it's how you treat, interact, and pour your hearts into your projects. We admire that so much about you both.

Creative Team (Chanelle Smith-Walker, Hristina & Bryant Polk, Jessi Lancaster & Ally Rabon): Thank you to our incredible creative team for capturing our vision. Mixing food and lifestyle is not an easy task. Your creativity, dedication, and attention to detail brought this to life in ways we could have never imagined. Your work elevated this project, and we are truly grateful for your talent and passion.

Mike and Judy Gallagher: Everyone needs a Mike and Judy in their life. You are a pillar of support, presence, and understanding. You are a daily reminder to us of what a great marriage looks like. As we have become parents, you have also been a rock for Sutton and Rosie.

Emma Kate DiLello: It's been an honor to have you on our team and a part of our lives. There have been far too many long days during the course of this project that we wouldn't have survived without you.

Jordyn Miro Hughes: Thank you for styling our family and helping Rach feel confident during a season when things don't always fit according to plan. You are the Law to her Zendaya.

Lauren Tully: The unofficial momager of the Sullivans, you've always been a text or phone call away for any advice, stamp of approval, or final vote. Thank you for inspiring me to start sharing my life on social media. It truly changed the projection of our lives.

DK/Publishing team: A huge thank you to the DK team for your support and guidance throughout this entire process. Your expertise, patience, and attention to detail have been invaluable in bringing this project to life. We are grateful for your hard work and dedication to making this book the best it can be. It's been a true privilege to work with such a talented and passionate team.

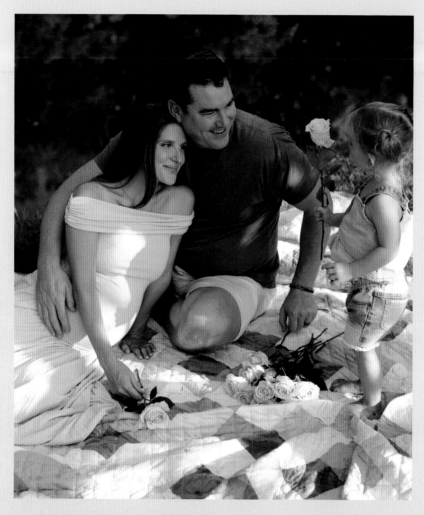

RACHAEL AND TOM SULLIVAN are *New York Times* bestselling authors and the couple behind the viral secret Instagram account Meals She Eats. Entertaining millions with their nourishing cooking and relatable lifestyle content, they have since appeared on *Good Morning America, the TODAY Show,* and *the Rachael Ray Show,* and have also been featured in numerous publications. Rachael and Tom reside in North Carolina with their daughters, Sutton and Rosie, and their perfect pup, Odin. Find them on Instagram and TikTok @MealsSheEats and @RachSullivan__. Their debut book, *Meals She Eats,* was published in 2023.